Living without a gallbladder can be a challenging adjustment, particularly when it comes to maintaining a balanced and nutritious diet. The gallbladder plays a crucial role in digestion by storing bile, which helps break down fats. When it's removed, your digestive system needs time and support to adapt to the changes. For those who choose a vegan lifestyle, this adjustment can seem even more daunting due to the specific dietary restrictions involved.

Welcome to the ***"No Gallbladder Diet Cookbook for Vegans: Rebalance and Revitalize for Sensitive Digestion After Gallbladder Removal with 110+ Recipes Over 90 Days."*** This book is designed to guide you through the process of adapting to life without a gallbladder while adhering to a vegan diet. It provides a comprehensive approach to nutrition that supports your digestive health and overall well-being.

Understanding Your New Dietary Needs

After gallbladder removal, your body no longer has a reservoir to store bile. This means that bile flows directly from your liver into your small intestine, which can lead to difficulties in digesting fats. Adapting your diet to these changes is essential to avoid discomfort and ensure you are absorbing the necessary nutrients from your food.

The Power of a Vegan Diet

A vegan diet, when properly managed, can be highly beneficial for those without a gallbladder. Plant-based foods tend to be easier to digest and are naturally lower in fat, making them ideal for sensitive digestion. This cookbook leverages the strengths of a vegan diet to help you rebalance and revitalize your digestive system.

What You Will Find in This Cookbook

This book is much more than just a collection of recipes; it is a comprehensive guide to navigating your post-surgery dietary needs. Inside, you will discover:

- ***Over 110 Vegan Recipes:*** Specially crafted to be gentle on your digestive system while providing all the essential nutrients. These recipes range from satisfying breakfasts and wholesome lunches to hearty dinners, snacks, and beverages.

- ***90-Day Meal Plan:*** A structured plan that helps you gradually adapt to your new dietary needs over three months. This plan ensures a balanced intake of nutrients while supporting your digestive health.

- ***Nutritional Guidance:*** Detailed nutritional information for each recipe to help you make informed choices and understand how different foods affect your digestion.

Adapting to life without a gallbladder while maintaining a vegan lifestyle requires dedication and the right knowledge. This cookbook is here to support you every step of the way. By following the recipes and advice within, you can look forward to improved digestion, enhanced energy levels, and a renewed sense of vitality.

Join us on this journey to better health. With the right dietary choices and a positive mindset, you can successfully manage your digestion without a gallbladder and continue to thrive on a vegan diet. Here's to rebalancing, revitalizing, and living your healthiest life!

I. Baked apples

Ingredient:

• 4 medium•sized apples (such as Gala, Fuji, or Honeycrisp)
• 1/4 cup rolled oats
• 2 tbsp chopped walnuts or pecans (optional)
• 2 tbsp maple syrup or agave nectar
• 1 tsp ground cinnamon
• 1/4 tsp ground nutmeg
• 1/4 cup unsweetened almond milk or oat milk

Instructions:
1. Preheat your oven to 375°F (190°C).

2. Wash the apples and use a sharp knife to cut off the top 1/4 of each apple. Scoop out the core and seeds, creating a small well in the center of each apple.

3. In a small bowl, mix together the rolled oats, chopped nuts (if using), maple syrup, cinnamon, and nutmeg.

4. Stuff the oat mixture into the hollowed•out centers of the apples, packing it in gently.

5. Place the stuffed apples in a baking dish and pour the almond or oat milk around the base of the apples.

6. Bake for 30•40 minutes, or until the apples are tender and the filling is lightly browned. Serve the baked apples warm, with the milk spooned over the top. Enjoy!

These baked apples are a great gallbladder•friendly dessert or snack, as they are low in fat and high in fiber from the apples and oats. The almond or oat milk provides a creamy, dairy•free element without adding any additional fat.

2. Applesauce

Ingredient:

• 6 medium apples, peeled, cored, and chopped (about 4 cups chopped)
• 1/2 cup water or unsweetened apple juice
• 2 tbsp maple syrup or honey (optional)
• 1 tsp ground cinnamon
• 1/4 tsp ground nutmeg

Instructions:

1. In a medium saucepan, combine the chopped apples and water or apple juice.

2. Bring the mixture to a boil over medium•high heat, then reduce the heat to low, cover, and simmer for 15•20 minutes, stirring occasionally, until the apples are very soft.

3. Remove the saucepan from the heat and let the apple mixture cool slightly.

4. Using a potato masher or an immersion blender, mash or blend the apples until you reach your desired consistency, whether chunky or smooth.

5. Stir in the maple syrup or honey (if using), cinnamon, and nutmeg. Taste and adjust seasonings as needed.

6. Serve the applesauce warm or chilled. It can be stored in an airtight container in the refrigerator for up to 1 week.

This homemade applesauce is a great gallbladder•friendly option as it is low in fat and high in fiber from the apples. The cinnamon and nutmeg add warmth and flavor without the need for additional sweeteners. Enjoy this applesauce on its own or use it as a topping for oatmeal, pancakes, or other dishes.

3. Bananas

Ingredient:

- 3 ripe bananas, frozen
- 1/4 cup unsweetened almond milk (or other plant•based milk)
- 1 tsp vanilla extract (optional)

Instructions:

1. Peel the ripe bananas and cut them into chunks. Place the banana chunks in a freezer•safe container and freeze for at least 2 hours, or until completely frozen.

2. Once the banana chunks are frozen, add them to a high•speed blender or food processor.

3. Pour in the unsweetened almond milk and add the vanilla extract (if using).

4. Blend the ingredients together, stopping to scrape down the sides as needed, until the mixture is smooth and creamy, with a soft•serve ice cream•like texture.

5. Serve the banana nice cream immediately, or transfer it to an airtight container and freeze for 30•60 minutes for a firmer consistency.

This recipe is perfect for those without a gallbladder because it's:

- Vegan • contains no dairy or animal products
- Low in fat • the only fat comes from the small amount of plant•based milk
- Easy to digest • bananas are gentle on the digestive system

You can enjoy this banana nice cream on its own or top it with fresh fruit, nuts, or a drizzle of nut butter for added nutrition and flavor. It's a delicious and healthy frozen treat that's easy on the gallbladder.

4. Berries (blueberries, raspberries, etc.)

Ingredient:

- 1/4 cup chia seeds
- 1 cup unsweetened almond milk (or other plant•based milk)
- 1 cup mixed berries (such as blueberries, raspberries, and/or blackberries)
- 1•2 tbsp maple syrup or honey (optional)

Instructions:

1. In a medium bowl, whisk together the chia seeds and almond milk until well combined.

2. Cover the bowl and refrigerate for at least 30 minutes, or up to overnight, stirring occasionally, until the mixture has thickened to a pudding•like consistency.

3. Once the chia pudding has thickened, stir in the mixed berries. If desired, drizzle in 1•2 tablespoons of maple syrup or honey to sweeten the pudding.

4. Divide the berry chia pudding into individual serving bowls or jars.

5. Refrigerate the pudding for at least 30 minutes before serving to allow the flavors to meld.

This berry chia pudding is a great option for those without a gallbladder because:

- It's vegan and dairy•free, making it easy to digest.
- The chia seeds provide fiber and protein without being too heavy on the gallbladder.
- The berries are low in fat and high in antioxidants, which can be beneficial for overall health.
- The maple syrup or honey is optional, so you can adjust the sweetness to your preference.

You can enjoy this berry chia pudding on its own or topped with additional fresh berries, nuts, or a sprinkle of cinnamon. It's a healthy, satisfying, and gallbladder•friendly treat.

5. Oranges

Ingredient:

• 3 medium oranges, peeled and segmented
• 4 cups mixed greens (such as spinach, arugula, or kale)
• 1 avocado, diced
• 1/4 cup toasted slivered almonds or chopped walnuts
• Orange Vinaigrette:
  • 1/4 cup fresh orange juice
  • 2 tbsp olive oil
  • 1 tbsp apple cider vinegar
  • 1 tsp Dijon mustard
  • 1 tsp maple syrup or honey (optional)
  • Salt and pepper to taste

Instructions:

1. In a large salad bowl, combine the orange segments, mixed greens, diced avocado, and toasted nuts.

2. In a small bowl or jar, whisk together the ingredients for the orange vinaigrette until well combined.

3. Drizzle the orange vinaigrette over the salad and gently toss to coat.

4. Serve the orange salad immediately.

This orange salad is a great option for those without a gallbladder because:

• The oranges are low in fat and high in vitamin C, which can be beneficial for overall health.
• The avocado provides healthy fats without being too heavy on the digestive system.
• The greens and nuts add fiber and nutrients without being too difficult to digest.
• The simple vinaigrette dressing is light and easy to digest, with no heavy creams or oils.

You can adjust the ingredients to your taste, such as adding more or less nuts, or using a different type of greens. This orange salad makes a refreshing and nourishing meal or side dish that is gentle on the gallbladder.

6. Grapefruit

Ingredient:

• 2 medium grapefruits, peeled and segmented
• 4 cups mixed greens (such as spinach, arugula, or kale)
• 1 avocado, diced
• 1/4 cup toasted slivered almonds or chopped walnuts
• Grapefruit Vinaigrette:
  • 1/4 cup fresh grapefruit juice
  • 2 tbsp olive oil
  • 1 tbsp apple cider vinegar
  • 1 tsp Dijon mustard
  • 1 tsp maple syrup or honey (optional)
  • Salt and pepper to taste

Instructions:

1. In a large salad bowl, combine the grapefruit segments, mixed greens, diced avocado, and toasted nuts.

2. In a small bowl or jar, whisk together the ingredients for the grapefruit vinaigrette until well combined.

3. Drizzle the grapefruit vinaigrette over the salad and gently toss to coat.

4. Serve the grapefruit salad immediately.

This grapefruit salad is a great option for those without a gallbladder because:

• The grapefruits are low in fat and high in vitamin C, which can be beneficial for overall health.
• The avocado provides healthy fats without being too heavy on the digestive system.
• The greens and nuts add fiber and nutrients without being too difficult to digest.
• The simple vinaigrette dressing is light and easy to digest, with no heavy creams or oils.

You can adjust the ingredients to your taste, such as adding more or less nuts, or using a different type of greens. This grapefruit salad makes a refreshing and nourishing meal or side dish that is gentle on the gallbladder.

7. Melons

Ingredient:

• 1 medium cantaloupe or honeydew melon, cut into 1•inch cubes
• Lime wedges (optional)

Instructions:

1. Preheat your grill or grill pan to medium•high heat.

2. Thread the melon cubes onto skewers, leaving a little space between each cube.

3. Grill the melon skewers for 2•3 minutes per side, or until you see grill marks and the melon is slightly softened.

4. Carefully remove the grilled melon skewers from the grill and transfer them to a serving platter.

5. Serve the grilled melon skewers immediately, with lime wedges on the side for guests to squeeze over the top if desired.

This grilled melon skewers recipe is a great option for those without a gallbladder because:

• Melons are low in fat and easy to digest, making them gentle on the digestive system.
• Grilling the melon adds a nice caramelized flavor without adding any heavy sauces or oils.
• The simple preparation allows the natural sweetness of the melon to shine.
• Serving the skewers with lime wedges provides a refreshing, acidic contrast that can aid digestion.

You can use any type of melon you prefer, such as cantaloupe, honeydew, or watermelon. The grilled melon skewers make a great appetizer, side dish, or even a light and healthy dessert option for those with gallbladder concerns.

8. Baked potatoes

Ingredient:

• 4 medium•sized russet potatoes
• 1/4 cup unsweetened almond milk (or other plant•based milk)
• 1/2 cup shredded vegan cheddar cheese (or other vegan cheese)
• 2 tablespoons chopped chives
• 1/4 teaspoon salt
• 1/8 teaspoon black pepper

Instructions:

1. Preheat your oven to 400°F (200°C).

2. Wash the potatoes and prick them several times with a fork. Place the potatoes directly on the oven rack and bake for 50•60 minutes, or until they are tender when pierced with a fork.

3. Remove the potatoes from the oven and let them cool for 10 minutes. Cut each potato in half lengthwise.

4. Carefully scoop the flesh out of the potato skins, leaving a thin layer of potato attached to the skin to help it hold its shape.

5. In a medium bowl, mash the potato flesh with the almond milk until smooth and creamy.

6. Stir in the shredded vegan cheese, chopped chives, salt, and black pepper until well combined.

7. Spoon the potato mixture back into the potato skins, dividing it evenly among the 8 halves.

8. Place the stuffed potato skins on a baking sheet and bake for an additional 15•20 minutes, or until the cheese is melted and the tops are lightly browned. Serve the twice•baked potatoes warm, garnished with extra chives if desired.

These vegan twice•baked potatoes are a great option for those without a gallbladder because:

• The potatoes are a gentle, low•fat carbohydrate source.
• The plant•based milk and cheese provide creaminess without being too heavy.
• The chives add flavor without being overly rich or spicy.

9. Boiled potatoes

Ingredient:

• 3 lbs (1.4 kg) Yukon Gold or Russet potatoes, peeled and cut into 1•inch cubes
• 1/2 cup (120 ml) unsweetened almond milk (or other plant•based milk)
• 2 tbsp (30 ml) vegan butter (optional)
• 1 tsp (5 ml) salt
• 1/4 tsp (1.25 ml) ground black pepper

Instructions:

1. Place the cubed potatoes in a large pot and cover with cold water. Bring to a boil over high heat.

2. Reduce the heat to medium•low and simmer the potatoes for 15•20 minutes, or until they are very tender when pierced with a fork.

3. Drain the potatoes in a colander and return them to the pot.

4. Add the almond milk and vegan butter (if using) to the potatoes. Use a potato masher or an electric hand mixer to mash the potatoes until smooth and creamy.

5. Stir in the salt and black pepper until well combined.

6. Taste and adjust seasoning as needed. Add more almond milk if you prefer a thinner consistency.

7. Serve the vegan boiled potato mash warm, garnished with chopped chives or parsley if desired.

This boiled potato mash is a great option for those without a gallbladder because:

• Boiling the potatoes is a gentle cooking method that preserves their nutrients.
• The plant•based milk and optional vegan butter provide creaminess without being too heavy.
• The simple seasoning of salt and pepper allows the natural potato flavor to shine.

Enjoy this comforting and easy•to•digest vegan potato mash as a side dish or as a base for other gallbladder•friendly toppings.

10. Tabbouleh (bulgur wheat salad)

Ingredient:

- 1 cup (170g) cooked bulgur wheat
- 1 cup (150g) diced tomatoes
- 1 cup (30g) chopped fresh parsley
- 1/2 cup (25g) chopped fresh mint
- 1/4 cup (40g) diced cucumber
- 2 tablespoons (30ml) lemon juice
- 2 tablespoons (30ml) olive oil
- 1 clove garlic, minced
- 1/4 teaspoon (1.25ml) salt
- 1/8 teaspoon (0.6ml) black pepper

Instructions:

1. Cook the bulgur wheat according to package instructions. Fluff with a fork and let cool.

2. In a large bowl, combine the cooked and cooled bulgur wheat, diced tomatoes, chopped parsley, chopped mint, and diced cucumber.

3. In a small bowl, whisk together the lemon juice, olive oil, minced garlic, salt, and black pepper.

4. Pour the dressing over the tabbouleh salad and toss gently to coat.

5. Refrigerate the tabbouleh for at least 30 minutes to allow the flavors to meld.

6. Serve chilled or at room temperature.

This vegan tabbouleh is a great option for those without a gallbladder because:

- Bulgur wheat is a whole grain that is easy to digest and low in fat.
- The fresh herbs, vegetables, and lemon juice provide flavor without being too heavy.
- The olive oil is a healthy fat that is gentle on the digestive system.
- The simple dressing is light and won't overwhelm the delicate flavors.

Tabbouleh makes a refreshing and nutritious side dish or light main course. Enjoy this gallbladder•friendly version as part of a balanced, plant•based diet.

II. Minestrone Soup

Ingredient:

• 1 tablespoon olive oil
• 1 onion, diced
• 3 cloves garlic, minced
• 2 carrots, peeled and diced
• 2 stalks celery, diced
• 1 zucchini, diced
• 1 (15 oz) can diced tomatoes
• 4 cups low•sodium vegetable broth
• 1 (15 oz) can kidney beans, rinsed and drained
• 1 cup cooked elbow macaroni
• 2 cups chopped kale or spinach
• 1 teaspoon dried oregano
• 1/2 teaspoon dried basil
• Salt and pepper to taste

Instructions:

1. In a large pot, heat the olive oil over medium heat. Add the onion and sauté for 3•4 minutes until translucent.

2. Add the garlic, carrots, celery, and zucchini. Sauté for an additional 5 minutes.

3. Pour in the diced tomatoes and vegetable broth. Bring the soup to a boil.

4. Reduce the heat to low and stir in the kidney beans, cooked macaroni, kale/spinach, oregano, and basil.

5. Simmer the soup for 10•15 minutes, until the vegetables are tender.

6. Season with salt and pepper to taste.

7. Serve the minestrone soup hot, garnished with extra chopped parsley if desired.

This vegan minestrone soup is a great option for those without a gallbladder because:

• It's low in fat and high in fiber from the vegetables and beans.
• The broth•based soup is easy to digest and won't overload the digestive system.
• The herbs and spices add flavor without being too heavy or rich.
• The inclusion of whole grains (macaroni) provides complex carbohydrates.

12. Vegetable Lentil Soup

Ingredient:

- 1 tablespoon olive oil
- 1 onion, diced
- 3 cloves garlic, minced
- 2 carrots, peeled and diced
- 2 stalks celery, diced
- 1 cup brown or green lentils, rinsed
- 4 cups low•sodium vegetable broth
- 1 (15 oz) can diced tomatoes
- 2 cups chopped kale or spinach
- 1 teaspoon dried thyme
- 1 teaspoon dried oregano
- Salt and pepper to taste

Instructions:

1. In a large pot, heat the olive oil over medium heat. Add the diced onion and sauté for 3•4 minutes until translucent.

2. Add the minced garlic, diced carrots, and diced celery. Sauté for an additional 5 minutes.

3. Stir in the rinsed lentils, vegetable broth, and diced tomatoes. Bring the soup to a boil.

4. Reduce the heat to low, cover the pot, and simmer for 20•25 minutes, or until the lentils are tender.

5. Stir in the chopped kale or spinach, dried thyme, and dried oregano. Cook for an additional 5 minutes.

6. Season the soup with salt and pepper to taste. Serve the vegetable lentil soup hot, garnished with extra chopped parsley if desired.

This vegan vegetable lentil soup is a great option for those without a gallbladder because:

- Lentils are a low•fat, high•fiber legume that is easy to digest.
- The vegetables provide a variety of nutrients without being too heavy.
- The broth•based soup is gentle on the digestive system.
- The herbs and spices add flavor without being overly rich or spicy.

13. Tomato Basil Soup

Ingredient:

- 1 tablespoon olive oil
- 1 onion, diced
- 3 cloves garlic, minced
- 1 (28 oz) can diced tomatoes
- 2 cups low•sodium vegetable broth
- 1/4 cup fresh basil leaves, chopped
- 1 teaspoon dried oregano
- 1/4 teaspoon red pepper flakes (optional)
- Salt and black pepper to taste
- 1/2 cup unsweetened almond milk (or other plant•based milk)

Instructions:

1. In a large pot, heat the olive oil over medium heat. Add the diced onion and sauté for 3•4 minutes until translucent.

2. Add the minced garlic and sauté for an additional minute, until fragrant.

3. Pour in the canned diced tomatoes and vegetable broth. Bring the soup to a simmer.

4. Stir in the chopped fresh basil, dried oregano, and red pepper flakes (if using). Season with salt and black pepper to taste.

5. Reduce the heat to low and let the soup simmer for 10•15 minutes, allowing the flavors to meld.

6. Remove the pot from the heat and carefully blend the soup using an immersion blender or transfer it to a regular blender in batches.

7. Once the soup is blended to your desired consistency, stir in the unsweetened almond milk.

8. Taste and adjust seasoning as needed. Serve the vegan tomato basil soup hot, garnished with extra fresh basil leaves if desired.

This tomato basil soup is a great option for those without a gallbladder because:

- The tomatoes and basil provide flavor without being too heavy or rich.
- The almond milk adds creaminess without using heavy cream.
- The simple ingredients are easy to digest and gentle on the digestive system.

14. Butternut Squash Soup

Ingredient:

- 1 medium butternut squash, peeled, seeded, and cubed (about 4 cups)
- 1 tablespoon olive oil
- 1 onion, diced
- 3 cloves garlic, minced
- 4 cups low•sodium vegetable broth
- 1 cup unsweetened almond milk
- 1 teaspoon ground cumin
- 1/2 teaspoon ground cinnamon
- 1/4 teaspoon ground nutmeg
- Salt and black pepper to taste
- Chopped fresh parsley for garnish (optional)

Instructions:

1. In a large pot or Dutch oven, heat the olive oil over medium heat. Add the diced onion and sauté for 3•4 minutes until translucent.

2. Add the minced garlic and sauté for an additional minute, until fragrant.

3. Add the cubed butternut squash and vegetable broth to the pot. Bring the mixture to a boil.

4. Reduce the heat to low, cover the pot, and simmer for 20•25 minutes, or until the squash is very tender.

5. Remove the pot from the heat and use an immersion blender to puree the soup until smooth. Alternatively, you can transfer the soup to a regular blender and blend in batches.

6. Stir in the unsweetened almond milk, ground cumin, ground cinnamon, and ground nutmeg. Season with salt and black pepper to taste.

7. Return the soup to low heat and simmer for an additional 5 minutes to allow the flavors to meld. Serve the butternut squash soup hot, garnished with chopped fresh parsley if desired.

This vegan butternut squash soup is a great option for those without a gallbladder because:

- Butternut squash is low in fat and easy to digest.
- The almond milk provides creaminess without being too heavy.

15. Miso Soup with Tofu and Seaweed

Ingredient:

• 4 cups low•sodium vegetable broth
• 2 tablespoons white or yellow miso paste
• 1 block firm or extra•firm tofu, cubed
• 1 cup thinly sliced shiitake mushrooms
• 1 cup chopped spinach or kale
• 2 tablespoons dried wakame seaweed (or other seaweed)
• 2 green onions, thinly sliced
• 1 teaspoon grated fresh ginger (optional)
• Salt and pepper to taste

Instructions:

1. In a medium saucepan, bring the vegetable broth to a gentle simmer over medium heat.

2. In a small bowl, whisk together the miso paste with a few tablespoons of the hot broth until smooth.

3. Carefully pour the miso mixture back into the saucepan with the broth, whisking to combine.

4. Add the cubed tofu, sliced shiitake mushrooms, chopped spinach/kale, and dried wakame seaweed to the broth. Simmer for 5•7 minutes, until the vegetables are tender.

5. Remove the soup from the heat and stir in the sliced green onions and grated ginger (if using).

6. Taste the soup and adjust seasoning with salt and pepper as needed.

7. Serve the miso soup hot, garnished with extra green onions if desired.

This vegan miso soup is a great option for those without a gallbladder because:

• Miso paste is a fermented soy product that is easy to digest.
• Tofu provides protein without being too heavy on the digestive system.
• Seaweed and leafy greens add nutrients without being too fibrous.
• The simple broth•based soup is gentle on the gallbladder.

16. Black Bean Soup

Ingredient:

- 1 tablespoon olive oil
- 1 onion, diced
- 3 cloves garlic, minced
- 2 carrots, peeled and diced
- 2 stalks celery, diced
- 2 (15 oz) cans black beans, rinsed and drained
- 4 cups low•sodium vegetable broth
- 1 (15 oz) can diced tomatoes
- 1 teaspoon ground cumin
- 1 teaspoon dried oregano
- 1/4 teaspoon cayenne pepper (optional)
- Salt and black pepper to taste
- Chopped cilantro for garnish (optional)

Instructions:

1. In a large pot or Dutch oven, heat the olive oil over medium heat. Add the diced onion and sauté for 3•4 minutes until translucent.

2. Add the minced garlic, diced carrots, and diced celery. Sauté for an additional 5 minutes.

3. Stir in the rinsed and drained black beans, vegetable broth, and diced tomatoes.

4. Add the ground cumin, dried oregano, and cayenne pepper (if using). Season with salt and black pepper to taste.

5. Bring the soup to a simmer and let it cook for 15•20 minutes, allowing the flavors to meld.

6. Using an immersion blender or regular blender, puree about half of the soup to thicken the consistency, leaving some whole beans intact.

7. Taste and adjust seasoning as needed. Serve the black bean soup hot, garnished with chopped cilantro if desired.

Enjoy this nourishing and gallbladder•friendly black bean soup as a main dish or side.

17. Potato Leek Soup

Ingredient:

- 1 tablespoon olive oil
- 2 leeks, white and light green parts only, thinly sliced
- 3 cloves garlic, minced
- 3 medium Yukon Gold potatoes, peeled and diced
- 4 cups low•sodium vegetable broth
- 1 cup unsweetened almond milk
- 1 teaspoon dried thyme
- Salt and white pepper to taste
- Chopped chives for garnish (optional)

Instructions:

1. In a large pot or Dutch oven, heat the olive oil over medium heat. Add the sliced leeks and sauté for 5•7 minutes, until softened.

2. Add the minced garlic and sauté for an additional minute, until fragrant.

3. Add the diced potatoes and vegetable broth to the pot. Bring the mixture to a boil.

4. Reduce the heat to low, cover the pot, and simmer for 20•25 minutes, or until the potatoes are very tender.

5. Remove the pot from the heat and use an immersion blender to puree the soup until smooth. Alternatively, you can transfer the soup to a regular blender and blend in batches.

6. Stir in the unsweetened almond milk and dried thyme. Season with salt and white pepper to taste.

7. Return the soup to low heat and simmer for an additional 5 minutes to allow the flavors to meld.

8. Serve the potato leek soup hot, garnished with chopped chives if desired.

Enjoy this nourishing and gallbladder•friendly potato leek soup as a comforting main dish or starter.

18. Chickpea and Spinach Stew

Ingredient:

- 1 tablespoon olive oil
- 1 onion, diced
- 3 cloves garlic, minced
- 2 carrots, peeled and diced
- 2 (15 oz) cans chickpeas, rinsed and drained
- 1 (15 oz) can diced tomatoes
- 4 cups low•sodium vegetable broth
- 2 cups fresh spinach, chopped
- 1 teaspoon ground cumin
- 1 teaspoon dried oregano
- Salt and black pepper to taste
- Chopped parsley for garnish (optional)

Instructions:

1. In a large pot or Dutch oven, heat the olive oil over medium heat. Add the diced onion and sauté for 3•4 minutes until translucent.

2. Add the minced garlic and diced carrots. Sauté for an additional 5 minutes.

3. Stir in the rinsed and drained chickpeas, diced tomatoes, and vegetable broth.

4. Add the ground cumin, dried oregano, and season with salt and black pepper to taste.

5. Bring the stew to a simmer and let it cook for 15•20 minutes, allowing the flavors to meld.

6. Stir in the chopped fresh spinach and cook for an additional 5 minutes, until the spinach is wilted.

7. Taste and adjust seasoning as needed.

8. Serve the chickpea and spinach stew hot, garnished with chopped parsley if desired.

Enjoy this nourishing and gallbladder•friendly chickpea and spinach stew as a main dish or side.

19. Curried Cauliflower Soup

Ingredient:

- 1 tablespoon olive oil
- 1 onion, diced
- 3 cloves garlic, minced
- 1 head of cauliflower, cut into florets (about 4 cups)
- 4 cups low•sodium vegetable broth
- 1 cup unsweetened almond milk
- 2 teaspoons curry powder
- 1 teaspoon ground cumin
- 1/4 teaspoon ground turmeric
- Salt and black pepper to taste
- Chopped cilantro for garnish (optional)

Instructions:

1. In a large pot or Dutch oven, heat the olive oil over medium heat. Add the diced onion and sauté for 3•4 minutes until translucent.

2. Add the minced garlic and sauté for an additional minute, until fragrant.

3. Add the cauliflower florets and vegetable broth to the pot. Bring the mixture to a boil.

4. Reduce the heat to low, cover the pot, and simmer for 20•25 minutes, or until the cauliflower is very tender.

5. Remove the pot from the heat and use an immersion blender to puree the soup until smooth. Alternatively, you can transfer the soup to a regular blender and blend in batches.

6. Stir in the unsweetened almond milk, curry powder, ground cumin, and ground turmeric. Season with salt and black pepper to taste.

7. Return the soup to low heat and simmer for an additional 5 minutes to allow the flavors to meld.

8. Serve the curried cauliflower soup hot, garnished with chopped cilantro if desired.

Enjoy this nourishing and gallbladder•friendly curried cauliflower soup as a comforting main dish or starter.

20. Vegetable and Quinoa Stew

Ingredient:

- 1 tablespoon olive oil
- 1 onion, diced
- 3 cloves garlic, minced
- 2 carrots, peeled and diced
- 2 stalks celery, diced
- 1 zucchini, diced
- 1 (15 oz) can diced tomatoes
- 4 cups low•sodium vegetable broth
- 1 cup uncooked quinoa, rinsed
- 1 (15 oz) can kidney beans, rinsed and drained
- 1 teaspoon dried thyme
- 1 teaspoon dried oregano
- Salt and black pepper to taste
- Chopped parsley for garnish (optional)

Instructions:

1. In a large pot or Dutch oven, heat the olive oil over medium heat. Add the diced onion and sauté for 3•4 minutes until translucent.

2. Add the minced garlic, diced carrots, diced celery, and diced zucchini. Sauté for an additional 5 minutes.

3. Stir in the diced tomatoes, vegetable broth, rinsed quinoa, and rinsed and drained kidney beans.

4. Add the dried thyme and dried oregano. Season with salt and black pepper to taste.

5. Bring the stew to a boil, then reduce the heat to low, cover the pot, and simmer for 20•25 minutes, or until the quinoa is cooked through and the vegetables are tender.

6. Taste and adjust seasoning as needed.

7. Serve the vegetable and quinoa stew hot, garnished with chopped parsley if desired.

Enjoy this nourishing and gallbladder•friendly vegetable and quinoa stew as a main dish or hearty side.

21. Stir•Fried Tofu with Vegetables

Ingredient:

• 1 block of extra•firm tofu, pressed and cubed
• 2 tbsp sesame oil
• 1 cup sliced mushrooms
• 1 cup chopped broccoli florets
• 1 cup sliced bell peppers
• 1 cup shredded cabbage
• 3 cloves garlic, minced
• 1 tbsp grated ginger
• 2 tbsp low•sodium soy sauce or tamari
• 1 tsp rice vinegar
• Salt and pepper to taste

Instructions:

1. In a large skillet or wok, heat the sesame oil over medium•high heat.

2. Add the cubed tofu and stir•fry for 3•4 minutes until lightly browned on all sides. Remove tofu from the pan and set aside.

3. In the same pan, add the mushrooms, broccoli, bell peppers, and cabbage. Stir•fry for 4•5 minutes until the vegetables are tender•crisp.

4. Add the garlic and ginger and cook for 1 minute, stirring constantly, until fragrant.

5. Return the tofu to the pan and add the soy sauce and rice vinegar. Toss everything together and cook for another 2•3 minutes.

6. Season with salt and pepper to taste.

7. Serve immediately over steamed brown rice or quinoa.

This dish is vegan, high in protein from the tofu, and low in fat and fiber, making it a great option for those without a gallbladder. The vegetables provide important nutrients without being too heavy on the digestive system.

22. Vegetable Stir•Fry

Ingredient:

• 2 tbsp sesame oil
• 1 cup sliced mushrooms
• 1 cup chopped broccoli florets
• 1 cup sliced carrots
• 1 cup snow peas or snap peas
• 1 cup shredded cabbage
• 3 cloves garlic, minced
• 1 tbsp grated ginger
• 2 tbsp low•sodium soy sauce or tamari
• 1 tsp rice vinegar
• Salt and pepper to taste

Instructions:

1. In a large skillet or wok, heat the sesame oil over medium•high heat.

2. Add the mushrooms, broccoli, carrots, snow peas, and cabbage. Stir•fry for 5•7 minutes, until the vegetables are tender•crisp.

3. Add the garlic and ginger and cook for 1 minute, stirring constantly, until fragrant.

4. Pour in the soy sauce and rice vinegar. Toss everything together and cook for another 2•3 minutes.

5. Season with salt and pepper to taste.

6. Serve immediately over steamed brown rice or quinoa.

This vegetable stir•fry is a great option for those without a gallbladder as it is low in fat and high in fiber, vitamins, and minerals. The variety of vegetables provides a range of nutrients while being easy to digest. You can adjust the vegetables based on your preferences or what's in season. Enjoy this flavorful and healthy dish!

23. Eggplant Parmesan (using vegan cheese)

Ingredient:

• 2 medium eggplants, sliced into 1/2•inch thick rounds
• 1 cup unsweetened almond milk
• 1 cup gluten•free breadcrumbs or panko
• 1 cup grated vegan parmesan cheese (such as Violife or Follow Your Heart)
• 1 jar (24 oz) marinara sauce
• 1 cup shredded vegan mozzarella cheese (such as Daiya or Miyoko's)
• Fresh basil leaves, for garnish

Instructions:

1. Preheat your oven to 375°F (190°C). Line a baking sheet with parchment paper.

2. Dip the eggplant slices in the almond milk, then dredge them in the breadcrumbs, pressing to help them adhere.

3. Arrange the breaded eggplant slices in a single layer on the prepared baking sheet. Bake for 20•25 minutes, flipping halfway, until golden brown.

4. Spread 1/2 cup of the marinara sauce in the bottom of a 9x13•inch baking dish. Arrange the baked eggplant slices in a single layer over the sauce.

5. Top the eggplant with the remaining marinara sauce, then sprinkle with the vegan parmesan and mozzarella cheeses.

6. Bake for 20•25 minutes, or until the cheese is melted and bubbly.

7. Remove from the oven and let cool for 5 minutes. Garnish with fresh basil leaves before serving.

This vegan eggplant parmesan dish is a delicious and satisfying option for those without a gallbladder. The eggplant is a low•fat, high•fiber vegetable, and the vegan cheeses are easy to digest. Serve this dish with a side salad or steamed vegetables for a complete and balanced meal.

24. Spaghetti with Marinara Sauce

Ingredient:

• 8 oz whole wheat or gluten•free spaghetti
• 1 tbsp olive oil
• 1 onion, diced
• 3 cloves garlic, minced
• 1 (28 oz) can crushed tomatoes
• 2 tbsp tomato paste
• 1 tsp dried oregano
• 1 tsp dried basil
• 1/4 tsp red pepper flakes (optional)
• Salt and pepper to taste
• Freshly chopped parsley for garnish (optional)

Instructions:

1. Bring a large pot of salted water to a boil. Cook the spaghetti according to package instructions until al dente. Drain and set aside.

2. In a large skillet, heat the olive oil over medium heat. Add the diced onion and sauté for 5•7 minutes until translucent.

3. Add the minced garlic and cook for 1 minute, until fragrant.

4. Pour in the crushed tomatoes and tomato paste. Stir to combine.

5. Add the dried oregano, basil, and red pepper flakes (if using). Season with salt and pepper to taste.

6. Simmer the sauce for 15•20 minutes, stirring occasionally, until thickened.

7. Add the cooked spaghetti to the sauce and toss to coat.

8. Serve the spaghetti with marinara sauce, garnished with freshly chopped parsley if desired.

This spaghetti with marinara sauce is a simple, yet flavorful dish that is easy on the digestive system. The whole wheat or gluten•free pasta provides fiber, while the tomato•based sauce is low in fat and easy to digest. Enjoy this comforting and satisfying meal!

25. Zucchini Noodles with Pesto

Ingredient:

- 3 medium zucchini, spiralized or julienned into noodles
- 1/2 cup basil pesto (store•bought or homemade)
- 1/4 cup toasted pine nuts
- 2 tbsp grated vegan parmesan cheese (optional)
- Salt and pepper to taste

For the Basil Pesto:
- 2 cups fresh basil leaves
- 1/4 cup pine nuts
- 2 cloves garlic
- 1/4 cup olive oil
- 2 tbsp lemon juice
- 1/4 cup grated vegan parmesan cheese (optional)
- Salt and pepper to taste

Instructions:

1. If making homemade pesto, combine all the pesto ingredients in a food processor or blender and blend until smooth. Set aside.

2. Spiralize or julienne the zucchini into noodle•like strands.

3. In a large bowl, toss the zucchini noodles with the basil pesto until well coated.

4. Top the zucchini noodles with the toasted pine nuts and grated vegan parmesan cheese (if using).

5. Season with salt and pepper to taste.

6. Serve immediately, or refrigerate for up to 3 days.

This zucchini noodle dish is a great low•carb, low•fat, and high•fiber option for those without a gallbladder. The pesto adds flavor and healthy fats from the olive oil and pine nuts. You can adjust the amount of pesto to your liking, and the vegan parmesan cheese is optional if you prefer to keep it dairy•free.

26. Black Bean Tacos with Corn Tortillas

Ingredient:

- 1 (15 oz) can black beans, rinsed and drained
- 1 tbsp olive oil
- 1 onion, diced
- 2 cloves garlic, minced
- 1 tsp ground cumin
- 1 tsp chili powder
- 1/4 tsp smoked paprika
- Salt and pepper to taste
- 8·10 small corn tortillas
- 1 cup shredded cabbage or lettuce
- 1 avocado, sliced
- 1/4 cup chopped cilantro
- 1 lime, cut into wedges

Instructions:

1. In a medium skillet, heat the olive oil over medium heat. Add the diced onion and sauté for 5·7 minutes until translucent.

2. Add the minced garlic and cook for 1 minute, until fragrant.

3. Add the rinsed and drained black beans, cumin, chili powder, and smoked paprika. Stir to combine and cook for 5·7 minutes, mashing some of the beans with the back of a spoon to create a slightly chunky texture.

4. Season the black bean mixture with salt and pepper to taste.

5. Warm the corn tortillas according to package instructions.

6. To assemble the tacos, place a spoonful of the black bean mixture into each tortilla. Top with shredded cabbage or lettuce, sliced avocado, and chopped cilantro.

7. Serve the tacos with lime wedges for squeezing over the top.

These black bean tacos are a great option for those without a gallbladder as they are high in fiber, low in fat, and easy to digest. The corn tortillas are a gluten·free and gentle option for the digestive system. Enjoy this flavorful and satisfying meal!

27. Lentil Shepherd's Pie

Ingredient:

For the Lentil Filling:
• 1 cup dry brown or green lentils, rinsed
• 3 cups vegetable broth
• 1 onion, diced
• 2 carrots, peeled and diced
• 2 celery stalks, diced
• 3 cloves garlic, minced
• 1 tsp dried thyme
• 1 tsp dried rosemary
• 1 tbsp tomato paste
• Salt and pepper to taste

For the Mashed Potato Topping:
• 3 lbs Yukon Gold potatoes, peeled and cut into 1•inch cubes
• 1/2 cup unsweetened almond milk
• 2 tbsp olive oil
• Salt and pepper to taste

Instructions:

1. Preheat your oven to 375°F (190°C).

2. In a large pot, combine the lentils and vegetable broth. Bring to a boil, then reduce heat and simmer for 20•25 minutes, until the lentils are tender. Drain any excess liquid and set aside.

3. In a large skillet, sauté the onion, carrots, and celery in a bit of water or broth for 5•7 minutes, until softened. Add the garlic and cook for 1 minute more.

4. Stir in the cooked lentils, thyme, rosemary, tomato paste, and season with salt and pepper to taste.

5. Transfer the lentil mixture to a 9x13•inch baking dish.

6. In a large pot, cover the cubed potatoes with water and bring to a boil. Reduce heat and simmer for 15•20 minutes, until the potatoes are tender. Drain and return to the pot.

7. Mash the potatoes with the almond milk and olive oil until smooth and creamy. Season with salt and pepper.

8. Spread the mashed potatoes evenly over the lentil filling. Bake the shepherd's pie for 30•35 minutes, until the potatoes are lightly browned. Let cool for 5•10 minutes before serving.

This lentil shepherd's pie is a hearty and comforting dish that is perfect for those without a gallbladder. The lentils provide protein and fiber, while the mashed potatoes are easy to digest.

28. Veggie Burger on Whole Grain Bun

Ingredient:

For the Veggie Patties:
• 1 (15 oz) can black beans, rinsed and drained
• 1 cup cooked quinoa
• 1/2 cup rolled oats
• 1/2 cup finely chopped mushrooms
• 1/4 cup finely chopped onion
• 2 cloves garlic, minced
• 1 tsp ground cumin
• 1 tsp chili powder
• 1/4 tsp smoked paprika
• Salt and pepper to taste

For the Burger:
• 4 whole grain buns, toasted
• Lettuce leaves
• Sliced tomatoes
• Avocado slices (optional)

Instructions:

1. In a large bowl, mash the black beans with a fork or potato masher until slightly chunky.

2. Add the cooked quinoa, rolled oats, chopped mushrooms, onion, garlic, cumin, chili powder, and smoked paprika. Mix well until fully combined.

3. Season the veggie burger mixture with salt and pepper to taste.

4. Divide the mixture into 4 equal portions and shape them into patties, about 1/2 inch thick.

5. Heat a large non•stick skillet over medium heat. Cook the veggie patties for 3•4 minutes per side, until lightly browned and heated through.

6. Place each veggie patty on a toasted whole grain bun. Top with lettuce, sliced tomatoes, and avocado slices (if using). Serve the veggie burgers immediately.

These veggie burgers are a great option for those without a gallbladder as they are high in fiber, low in fat, and easy to digest. The whole grain buns provide additional fiber and nutrients. Feel free to customize the toppings to your liking.

29. Roasted Vegetable Pizza (with thin crust)

Ingredient:

For the Toppings:
- 1 cup sliced mushrooms
- 1 cup chopped bell peppers
- 1 cup chopped zucchini
- 1 cup chopped onion
- 2 cloves garlic, minced
- 2 tbsp olive oil
- Salt and pepper to taste
- 1 cup marinara sauce
- 1 cup shredded vegan mozzarella cheese

For the Crust:
- 1 cup whole wheat flour
- 1 cup all•purpose flour
- 1 tsp active dry yeast
- 1 tsp salt
- 3/4 cup warm water
- 1 tbsp olive oil

Instructions:

1. Preheat your oven to 450°F (230°C).

2. In a large bowl, combine the whole wheat flour, all•purpose flour, yeast, and salt. Add the warm water and olive oil, and mix until a dough forms.

3. Knead the dough on a lightly floured surface for 5•7 minutes, until smooth and elastic.

4. Roll or stretch the dough into a thin, round crust and place it on a baking sheet or pizza pan.

5. In a large bowl, toss the sliced mushrooms, bell peppers, zucchini, onion, and minced garlic with the 2 tbsp of olive oil. Season with salt and pepper.

6. Spread the marinara sauce evenly over the pizza crust, leaving a small border.

7. Arrange the roasted vegetables over the sauce, then sprinkle the shredded vegan mozzarella cheese on top.

8. Bake the pizza for 15•20 minutes, or until the crust is golden brown and the cheese is melted and bubbly. Let the pizza cool for 5 minutes before slicing and serving.

This roasted vegetable pizza with a thin, whole wheat crust is a great option for those without a gallbladder. The vegetables provide fiber and nutrients, while the vegan cheese is easy to digest. Enjoy this delicious and healthy pizza!

30. Cauliflower Steaks

Ingredient:

- 1 large head of cauliflower, cut into 1•inch thick slices (cauliflower "steaks")
- 2 tbsp olive oil
- 1 tsp garlic powder
- 1 tsp paprika
- 1/2 tsp salt
- 1/4 tsp black pepper

Instructions:

1. Preheat your oven to 400°F (200°C).

2. Lay the cauliflower steaks on a baking sheet lined with parchment paper.

3. In a small bowl, mix together the olive oil, garlic powder, paprika, salt, and black pepper.

4. Brush the seasoning mixture evenly over the top of the cauliflower steaks.

5. Bake for 20•25 minutes, flipping the steaks halfway, until the cauliflower is tender and lightly browned on the edges.

6. Serve the cauliflower steaks warm, garnished with fresh herbs if desired.

This recipe is vegan and does not contain any ingredients that would be problematic for those without a gallbladder. The cauliflower is a low•fat, low•fiber vegetable that is easy to digest. The simple seasoning adds flavor without any heavy sauces or oils.

31. Pasta Primavera

Ingredient:

- 8 oz whole wheat or gluten•free pasta
- 1 tbsp olive oil
- 1 cup sliced mushrooms
- 1 cup chopped broccoli florets
- 1 cup chopped zucchini
- 1 cup chopped bell pepper
- 3 cloves garlic, minced
- 1 tsp dried basil
- 1 tsp dried oregano
- 1/4 tsp red pepper flakes (optional)
- 1/4 cup unsweetened almond milk
- 2 tbsp nutritional yeast
- Salt and black pepper to taste

Instructions:

1. Bring a large pot of salted water to a boil. Cook the pasta according to package instructions until al dente. Drain and set aside.

2. In a large skillet, heat the olive oil over medium heat. Add the mushrooms, broccoli, zucchini, bell pepper, and garlic. Sauté for 5•7 minutes until the vegetables are tender•crisp.

3. Add the cooked pasta, basil, oregano, red pepper flakes (if using), almond milk, and nutritional yeast to the skillet. Toss everything together until well combined and heated through.

4. Season with salt and black pepper to taste.

5. Serve the Pasta Primavera warm, garnished with extra fresh herbs if desired.

This recipe is vegan and uses a variety of fresh vegetables that are easy to digest for those without a gallbladder. The whole wheat or gluten•free pasta provides fiber, while the almond milk and nutritional yeast add creaminess without any dairy products.

32. Quinoa Stuffed Bell Peppers

Ingredient:

• 4 medium bell peppers, halved lengthwise and seeds removed
• 1 cup cooked quinoa
• 1 (15 oz) can black beans, rinsed and drained
• 1 cup diced tomatoes
• 1/2 cup diced onion
• 2 cloves garlic, minced
• 1 tsp ground cumin
• 1 tsp dried oregano
• 1/4 tsp chili powder
• Salt and black pepper to taste
• 1/4 cup chopped fresh cilantro (optional)

Instructions:

1. Preheat your oven to 375°F (190°C).

2. Arrange the bell pepper halves in a baking dish or on a rimmed baking sheet.

3. In a medium bowl, combine the cooked quinoa, black beans, diced tomatoes, onion, garlic, cumin, oregano, and chili powder. Season with salt and black pepper to taste.

4. Spoon the quinoa mixture evenly into the bell pepper halves.

5. Cover the baking dish or sheet with foil and bake for 25•30 minutes, until the peppers are tender.

6. Remove the foil and bake for an additional 5•10 minutes, until the tops are lightly browned.

7. Garnish the stuffed peppers with fresh chopped cilantro, if desired.

8. Serve the Vegan Quinoa Stuffed Bell Peppers warm.

This recipe is vegan and uses a variety of fiber•rich, low•fat ingredients that are easy to digest for those without a gallbladder. The quinoa and black beans provide protein, while the bell peppers and other vegetables offer essential vitamins and minerals.

33. Brown Rice with Steamed Vegetables

Ingredient:

• 1 cup uncooked brown rice
• 2 cups low•sodium vegetable broth
• 1 cup broccoli florets
• 1 cup sliced carrots
• 1 cup chopped zucchini
• 1 cup sliced mushrooms
• 2 cloves garlic, minced
• 1 tbsp low•sodium soy sauce or tamari
• 1 tsp sesame oil (optional)
• Salt and pepper to taste

Instructions:

1. In a medium saucepan, combine the brown rice and vegetable broth. Bring to a boil, then reduce heat to low, cover, and simmer for 25•30 minutes, until the rice is tender and the liquid is absorbed.

2. While the rice is cooking, prepare the steamed vegetables. In a steamer basket or saucepan with a steamer insert, steam the broccoli, carrots, zucchini, and mushrooms for 5•7 minutes, until tender•crisp.

3. In a large bowl, combine the cooked brown rice, steamed vegetables, minced garlic, soy sauce, and sesame oil (if using). Toss gently to mix.

4. Season the brown rice and vegetable dish with salt and pepper to taste.

5. Serve the brown rice and steamed vegetables warm.

This brown rice and steamed vegetable dish is a great option for those without a gallbladder. The brown rice provides complex carbohydrates and fiber, while the steamed vegetables are low in fat and easy to digest. The soy sauce and sesame oil (if using) add flavor without being too heavy on the digestive system.

You can adjust the vegetables based on your preferences or what's in season. This dish is a simple, yet nutritious and satisfying meal.

34. Vegan Paella

Ingredient:

- 1 cup short•grain brown rice
- 3 cups vegetable broth
- 1 tbsp olive oil
- 1 onion, diced
- 3 cloves garlic, minced
- 1 red bell pepper, diced
- 1 cup diced tomatoes
- 1 tsp smoked paprika
- 1 tsp dried thyme
- 1/2 tsp saffron threads (optional)
- 1 cup frozen peas
- 1 (15 oz) can chickpeas, rinsed and drained
- Salt and black pepper to taste
- Chopped parsley for garnish

Instructions:

1. In a large saucepan, bring the vegetable broth to a boil. Add the brown rice, cover, and reduce heat to low. Simmer for 30•35 minutes, until the rice is tender and the liquid is absorbed. Fluff with a fork and set aside.

2. In a large skillet or paella pan, heat the olive oil over medium heat. Add the onion and sauté for 3•4 minutes until translucent.

3. Add the garlic, bell pepper, diced tomatoes, smoked paprika, thyme, and saffron (if using). Cook for 5•7 minutes, stirring occasionally, until the vegetables are tender.

4. Stir in the cooked brown rice, frozen peas, and chickpeas. Season with salt and black pepper to taste.

5. Cook for an additional 5•10 minutes, stirring occasionally, until everything is heated through and the flavors have melded.

6. Serve the Vegan Paella hot, garnished with chopped parsley.

This recipe is vegan and uses ingredients that are easy to digest for those without a gallbladder, such as brown rice, vegetables, and legumes. The spices and herbs add flavor without any heavy sauces or oils.

35. Couscous Salad with Chickpeas

Ingredient:

- 1 cup dry couscous
- 1 cup boiling water
- 1 (15 oz) can chickpeas, rinsed and drained
- 1 cup diced cucumber
- 1 cup diced tomatoes
- 1/2 cup diced red onion
- 1/4 cup chopped fresh parsley
- 2 tbsp lemon juice
- 2 tbsp olive oil
- 1 tsp ground cumin
- 1/2 tsp ground coriander
- Salt and black pepper to taste

Instructions:

1. In a medium bowl, combine the dry couscous and boiling water. Cover and let sit for 5•10 minutes, until the couscous has absorbed all the water. Fluff with a fork.

2. Add the chickpeas, cucumber, tomatoes, red onion, and parsley to the cooked couscous. Toss to combine.

3. In a small bowl, whisk together the lemon juice, olive oil, cumin, and coriander. Season with salt and black pepper to taste.

4. Pour the dressing over the couscous salad and toss gently to coat everything evenly.

5. Refrigerate the Vegan Couscous Salad with Chickpeas for at least 30 minutes to allow the flavors to meld.

6. Serve chilled or at room temperature.

This recipe is vegan and uses ingredients that are easy to digest for those without a gallbladder, such as couscous, chickpeas, and fresh vegetables. The simple dressing adds flavor without any heavy oils or sauces.

36. Orzo with Roasted Vegetables

Ingredient:

• 1 cup dry orzo pasta
• 1 cup cubed butternut squash
• 1 cup chopped bell peppers
• 1 cup sliced mushrooms
• 1 cup chopped zucchini
• 1 onion, diced
• 3 cloves garlic, minced
• 2 tbsp olive oil
• 1 tsp dried thyme
• 1 tsp dried oregano
• Salt and pepper to taste
• 2 tbsp chopped fresh parsley (optional)

Instructions:

1. Preheat your oven to 400°F (200°C). Line a baking sheet with parchment paper.

2. In a large bowl, toss the cubed butternut squash, chopped bell peppers, sliced mushrooms, chopped zucchini, and diced onion with the olive oil, dried thyme, dried oregano, salt, and pepper.

3. Spread the vegetables in a single layer on the prepared baking sheet. Roast for 20•25 minutes, stirring halfway, until the vegetables are tender and lightly browned.

4. While the vegetables are roasting, cook the orzo according to the package instructions. Drain and set aside.

5. In a large bowl, combine the roasted vegetables and the cooked orzo. Toss to mix well.

6. Stir in the minced garlic and adjust the seasoning with additional salt and pepper, if desired.

7. Garnish the orzo with chopped fresh parsley, if using. Serve the orzo with roasted vegetables warm or at room temperature.

This orzo with roasted vegetables dish is a great option for those without a gallbladder. The orzo provides a source of complex carbohydrates, while the roasted vegetables are low in fat and high in fiber, vitamins, and minerals. The dish is easy to digest and provides a balanced and satisfying meal.

37. Soba Noodle Salad with Peanut Dressing

Ingredient:

• 8 oz soba noodles
• 1 cup shredded cabbage
• 1 cup shredded carrots
• 1 cup diced cucumber
• 1/2 cup chopped green onions
• 1/4 cup chopped fresh cilantro
• 2 tbsp toasted sesame seeds

For the Peanut Dressing:
• 1/4 cup creamy peanut butter
• 2 tbsp rice vinegar
• 2 tbsp low•sodium soy sauce
• 1 tbsp maple syrup
• 1 tbsp sesame oil
• 1 tsp grated fresh ginger
• 1•2 tbsp warm water to thin

Instructions:

1. Cook the soba noodles according to package instructions. Drain and rinse under cold water until cool. Set aside.

2. In a large bowl, combine the shredded cabbage, carrots, diced cucumber, green onions, and chopped cilantro. Add the cooked soba noodles and toss to mix.

3. In a small bowl, whisk together all the ingredients for the peanut dressing, adding warm water 1 tbsp at a time until the desired consistency is reached.

4. Pour the peanut dressing over the soba noodle salad and toss to coat everything evenly.

5. Sprinkle the toasted sesame seeds over the top.

6. Refrigerate the Vegan Soba Noodle Salad with Peanut Dressing for at least 30 minutes before serving to allow the flavors to meld.

This recipe is vegan and uses ingredients that are easy to digest for those without a gallbladder, such as soba noodles, vegetables, and a peanut•based dressing. The peanut butter provides protein, while the vegetables offer fiber and nutrients.

38. Vegan Mac and Cheese

Ingredient:

- 8 oz elbow macaroni or other small pasta shape
- 1 cup raw cashews, soaked in water for at least 4 hours or overnight
- 1 cup unsweetened almond milk
- 1/2 cup nutritional yeast
- 2 tbsp lemon juice
- 1 tsp Dijon mustard
- 1 tsp garlic powder
- 1/2 tsp onion powder
- 1/2 tsp salt
- 1/4 tsp black pepper

Instructions:

1. Cook the pasta according to package instructions. Drain and set aside.

2. Drain and rinse the soaked cashews. Add them to a high•speed blender along with the almond milk, nutritional yeast, lemon juice, Dijon mustard, garlic powder, onion powder, salt, and black pepper. Blend until smooth and creamy.

3. In a large saucepan, combine the cooked pasta and the cashew cheese sauce. Heat over medium, stirring frequently, until the sauce thickens and the pasta is heated through, about 5•7 minutes.

4. Serve the Vegan Mac and Cheese warm, garnished with chopped parsley or chives if desired.

This recipe is vegan and uses cashews and nutritional yeast to create a creamy, cheese•like sauce that is easy to digest for those without a gallbladder. The pasta provides complex carbohydrates, while the cashews offer healthy fats and protein.

39. Farro Risotto with Mushrooms

Ingredient:

- 1 cup dry farro
- 4 cups low•sodium vegetable broth
- 1 tbsp olive oil
- 1 onion, diced
- 8 oz sliced mushrooms
- 3 cloves garlic, minced
- 1 tsp dried thyme
- 1/4 cup dry white wine (optional)
- 1/4 cup grated vegan parmesan cheese (optional)
- Salt and pepper to taste
- Chopped fresh parsley for garnish (optional)

Instructions:

1. In a medium saucepan, bring the vegetable broth to a simmer and keep it warm over low heat.

2. In a large skillet or Dutch oven, heat the olive oil over medium heat. Add the diced onion and sauté for 5•7 minutes until translucent.

3. Add the sliced mushrooms and continue to sauté for 3•4 minutes, until the mushrooms are lightly browned.

4. Stir in the minced garlic and dried thyme, and cook for 1 minute until fragrant.

5. Add the dry farro to the skillet and stir to coat the grains with the oil and vegetables.

6. If using, pour in the white wine and let it simmer for 2•3 minutes, until the wine is mostly absorbed.

7. Ladle in the warm vegetable broth, about 1/2 cup at a time, stirring constantly until the liquid is absorbed before adding more. Continue this process for 25•30 minutes, until the farro is tender and has a creamy, risotto•like texture.

8. Remove the farro risotto from heat and stir in the grated vegan parmesan cheese, if using. Season with salt and pepper to taste. Serve the farro risotto warm, garnished with chopped fresh parsley, if desired.

This farro risotto with mushrooms is a great option for those without a gallbladder. Farro is a whole grain that is high in fiber and easy to digest, while the mushrooms provide additional nutrients and flavor. The dish is low in fat and can be made dairy•free by omitting the vegan parmesan cheese.

40. Spicy Thai Noodles

Ingredient:

• 8 oz rice noodles
• 2 tbsp coconut oil
• 3 cloves garlic, minced
• 1 tbsp grated fresh ginger
• 1 red bell pepper, thinly sliced
• 1 cup shredded cabbage
• 1 cup shredded carrots
• 2 green onions, sliced
• 1/4 cup chopped fresh cilantro
• 2 tbsp low•sodium soy sauce or tamari
• 1 tbsp lime juice
• 1•2 tsp red curry paste (start with 1 tsp for less heat)
• 1 tsp brown sugar
• Salt and black pepper to taste

Instructions:

1. Cook the rice noodles according to package instructions. Drain and rinse under cold water.

2. In a large skillet or wok, heat the coconut oil over medium heat. Add the minced garlic and grated ginger. Cook for 1 minute, stirring constantly, until fragrant.

3. Add the sliced red bell pepper, shredded cabbage, shredded carrots, and green onions. Sauté for 3•5 minutes, until the vegetables are tender•crisp.

4. Add the cooked rice noodles, soy sauce, lime juice, red curry paste, and brown sugar. Toss everything together until well combined and heated through.

5. Remove from heat and stir in the chopped fresh cilantro. Season with salt and black pepper to taste.

6. Serve the Spicy Thai Noodles warm, garnished with extra cilantro if desired.

This recipe is vegan and uses ingredients that are easy to digest for those without a gallbladder, such as rice noodles, vegetables, and a simple sauce made with coconut oil, soy sauce, and red curry paste.

41. Steamed Broccoli with Lemon

Ingredient:

- 1 lb broccoli florets
- 2 tbsp water
- 1 tbsp fresh lemon juice
- 1 tsp lemon zest
- 1/4 tsp salt
- 1/8 tsp black pepper

Instructions:

1. In a steamer basket set over a saucepan of simmering water, steam the broccoli florets for 5•7 minutes, until tender•crisp.

2. Transfer the steamed broccoli to a serving bowl.

3. In a small bowl, whisk together the lemon juice, lemon zest, salt, and black pepper.

4. Drizzle the lemon dressing over the steamed broccoli and toss gently to coat.

5. Serve the Steamed Broccoli with Lemon warm or at room temperature.

This recipe is vegan and uses simple, easy•to•digest ingredients. Broccoli is a low•fat, high•fiber vegetable that is generally well•tolerated by those without a gallbladder. The lemon juice and zest add flavor without any heavy sauces or oils.

This dish is a great side option that is light, refreshing, and easy on the digestive system. The steaming method helps to preserve the nutrients in the broccoli, while the lemon dressing provides a bright, tangy contrast.

42. Garlic Roasted Brussels Sprouts

Ingredient:

- 1 lb Brussels sprouts, trimmed and halved
- 2 tbsp olive oil
- 3 cloves garlic, minced
- 1 tsp dried thyme
- 1/2 tsp salt
- 1/4 tsp black pepper

Instructions:

1. Preheat your oven to 400°F (200°C). Line a baking sheet with parchment paper.

2. In a large bowl, toss the trimmed and halved Brussels sprouts with the olive oil, minced garlic, dried thyme, salt, and black pepper until the sprouts are evenly coated.

3. Spread the seasoned Brussels sprouts in a single layer on the prepared baking sheet.

4. Roast for 20•25 minutes, tossing halfway, until the Brussels sprouts are tender and lightly browned.

5. Serve the Garlic Roasted Brussels Sprouts warm, as a side dish.

This recipe is vegan and uses simple, easy•to•digest ingredients. Brussels sprouts are a low•fat, high•fiber vegetable that is generally well•tolerated by those without a gallbladder. The garlic and thyme add flavor without any heavy sauces or oils.

43. Coconut milk

Ingredient:

- 1 tbsp coconut oil
- 1 onion, diced
- 3 cloves garlic, minced
- 1 tbsp grated fresh ginger
- 2 tsp curry powder
- 1 tsp ground cumin
- 1 (13.5 oz) can full•fat coconut milk
- 1 cup diced tomatoes
- 1 cup cooked chickpeas
- Salt and black pepper to taste
- Chopped cilantro for garnish

Instructions:

1. In a large skillet, heat the coconut oil over medium heat. Add the onion and sauté for 3•4 minutes until translucent.

2. Add the garlic, ginger, curry powder, and cumin. Cook for 1 minute, stirring constantly.

3. Pour in the coconut milk and diced tomatoes. Bring to a simmer and add the chickpeas.

4. Simmer for 10•15 minutes, until the sauce has thickened. Season with salt and black pepper.

5. Serve the Coconut Milk Curry over steamed rice or quinoa, garnished with chopped cilantro.

These recipes use coconut milk, which is a dairy•free, low•lactose option that is generally well•tolerated by those without a gallbladder. The healthy fats and fiber in coconut milk can be beneficial for digestion.

44. Vegan cheeses

Ingredient:

• 1 cup raw cashews, soaked in water for at least 4 hours or overnight
• 1/2 cup unsweetened almond milk
• 2 tbsp lemon juice
• 1 tbsp nutritional yeast
• 1/2 tsp salt
• 1/4 tsp garlic powder

Instructions:
1. Drain and rinse the soaked cashews.

2. Add the cashews, almond milk, lemon juice, nutritional yeast, salt, and garlic powder to a high•speed blender. Blend until smooth and creamy.

3. Transfer the cheese mixture to a small bowl or ramekin and refrigerate for at least 2 hours before serving.

Nut•Free Vegan Cheese Sauce
Ingredients:
• 1 cup cooked white beans, drained and rinsed
• 1/2 cup unsweetened almond milk
• 2 tbsp nutritional yeast
• 1 tbsp lemon juice
• 1 tsp Dijon mustard
• 1/2 tsp garlic powder
• 1/4 tsp onion powder
• 1/4 tsp salt

Instructions:
1. Add all the ingredients to a high•speed blender and blend until smooth and creamy.

2. Transfer the cheese sauce to a saucepan and heat over medium, stirring frequently, until warmed through. Use the cheese sauce as a dip, topping, or in recipes that call for cheese.

Both of these vegan cheese recipes are nut•free and use simple, easy•to•digest ingredients that are suitable for those without a gallbladder, such as cashews, white beans, and nutritional yeast. They provide a creamy, cheese•like texture and flavor without any dairy products.

45. Vegan yogurts

Ingredient:

- 1 (13.5 oz) can full•fat coconut milk
- 2 tbsp unsweetened coconut meat (optional)
- 1 tbsp probiotic powder or 2•3 probiotic capsules

Instructions:

1. In a medium saucepan, heat the coconut milk over medium heat, stirring frequently, until it reaches 110°F•115°F on a food thermometer.

2. Remove the coconut milk from heat and let it cool to 100°F•105°F. This temperature range is important for the probiotics to activate.

3. If using, stir in the unsweetened coconut meat.

4. Add the probiotic powder or contents of the probiotic capsules and whisk thoroughly to combine.

5. Pour the mixture into a clean glass jar or container. Cover and place in a warm spot (around 100°F) for 6•8 hours, or until the yogurt has thickened to your desired consistency.

6. Once thickened, transfer the coconut milk yogurt to the refrigerator and chill for at least 4 hours before serving.

7. The yogurt will continue to thicken as it chills. Stir before serving.

This homemade coconut milk yogurt is dairy•free, vegan, and contains live active cultures that can be beneficial for digestion. The full•fat coconut milk provides healthy fats that are easy to digest for those without a gallbladder.

You can enjoy the coconut yogurt plain or top it with fresh fruit, nuts, granola, or a drizzle of maple syrup.

46. Veggie burgers

Ingredient:

- 1 (15 oz) can black beans, rinsed and drained
- 1 cup cooked quinoa
- 1/2 cup rolled oats
- 1/2 cup finely chopped mushrooms
- 1/2 cup grated carrot
- 1/4 cup finely chopped onion
- 2 cloves garlic, minced
- 1 tsp ground cumin
- 1 tsp smoked paprika
- 1/2 tsp dried thyme
- 1/4 tsp cayenne pepper (optional)
- Salt and black pepper to taste
- Whole wheat buns or lettuce wraps, for serving

Instructions:

1. In a large bowl, mash the black beans with a fork or potato masher, leaving some texture.

2. Add the cooked quinoa, rolled oats, chopped mushrooms, grated carrot, onion, garlic, cumin, smoked paprika, thyme, and cayenne (if using). Season with salt and black pepper.

3. Mix all the ingredients together until well combined.

4. Divide the mixture into 6•8 equal portions and shape them into patties, about 1/2 inch thick.

5. Heat a large non•stick skillet over medium heat. Cook the veggie patties for 3•4 minutes per side, until lightly browned and heated through.

6. Serve the Vegan Veggie Burgers on whole wheat buns or in lettuce wraps, with your favorite toppings like avocado, tomato, and onion.

This recipe is vegan and uses a variety of plant•based ingredients that are easy to digest for those without a gallbladder, such as black beans, quinoa, oats, and vegetables. The patties are baked instead of fried, making them a healthier option.

47. Vegan protein powder shakes

Ingredient:

- 1 cup unsweetened almond milk
- 2 tbsp peanut butter
- 1 scoop chocolate vegan protein powder
- 1 tbsp cocoa powder
- 1 tsp maple syrup (optional)
- Ice cubes

Instructions:

1. Add all the ingredients to a blender.

2. Blend on high speed until smooth and creamy.

3. Taste and adjust sweetness with maple syrup if desired.

4. Pour into a glass and enjoy!

This shake is a delicious way to get a boost of plant•based protein along with the classic flavor combination of chocolate and peanut butter. The almond milk provides a creamy base, while the peanut butter adds healthy fats and extra flavor. Feel free to adjust the amounts of any ingredients to suit your taste preferences.

48. Seitan

Ingredient:

• 1 lb seitan, cut into bite•sized pieces
• 2 tbsp soy sauce
• 1 tbsp rice vinegar
• 1 tsp sesame oil
• 2 cloves garlic, minced
• 1 inch ginger, grated
• 2 cups mixed veggies (e.g. broccoli, bell peppers, snap peas)
• Cooked rice or noodles, to serve

Instructions:

1. In a small bowl, whisk together the soy sauce, rice vinegar, and sesame oil. Set aside.

2. Heat a large skillet or wok over medium•high heat. Add the seitan pieces and stir•fry for 3•4 minutes until lightly browned.

3. Add the minced garlic and grated ginger to the pan. Stir•fry for 1 minute until fragrant.

4. Add the mixed vegetables to the pan. Stir•fry for 4•5 minutes until the vegetables are tender•crisp.

5. Pour the soy sauce mixture over the seitan and vegetables. Toss everything together and cook for 2•3 minutes, until the sauce has thickened slightly.

6. Serve the seitan stir•fry immediately over cooked rice or noodles.

This stir•fry is a quick and easy way to enjoy the savory, meaty texture of seitan with fresh vegetables and a flavorful sauce. Feel free to adjust the vegetable mix to your liking. Enjoy!

49. Vegetable soups

Ingredient:

- 1 onion, diced
- 3 carrots, diced
- 3 celery stalks, diced
- 3 cloves garlic, minced
- 1 can (14.5 oz) diced tomatoes
- 4 cups vegetable broth
- 1 can (15 oz) kidney beans, drained and rinsed
- 1 cup elbow macaroni
- 2 cups chopped kale or spinach
- Salt and pepper to taste

Instructions:

1. In a large pot or Dutch oven, sauté the onion, carrots, and celery in a bit of olive oil over medium heat for 5•7 minutes, until softened.

2. Add the minced garlic and cook for 1 minute more, until fragrant.

3. Pour in the can of diced tomatoes and the vegetable broth. Bring the soup to a simmer.

4. Add the kidney beans and the elbow macaroni. Cook for 8•10 minutes, until the pasta is tender.

5. Stir in the chopped kale or spinach and cook for 2•3 minutes more, until the greens are wilted.

6. Season the soup with salt and pepper to taste.

7. Ladle the minestrone soup into bowls and serve hot.

This hearty minestrone soup is packed with nutritious vegetables, beans, and pasta. It's a comforting and satisfying meatless meal. Feel free to adjust the vegetable mix or add any other favorite ingredients. Enjoy!

50. Lentil soups

Ingredient:

• 1 cup brown or green lentils, rinsed
• 6 cups low•sodium vegetable broth
• 1 onion, diced
• 2 carrots, peeled and diced
• 2 celery stalks, diced
• 3 cloves garlic, minced
• 1 tsp dried thyme
• 1 tsp dried oregano
• 1/2 tsp smoked paprika
• Salt and black pepper to taste
• Chopped parsley for garnish (optional)

Instructions:

1. In a large pot, combine the lentils and vegetable broth. Bring to a boil, then reduce heat and simmer for 15•20 minutes, until lentils are tender.

2. Add the onion, carrots, celery, garlic, thyme, oregano, and smoked paprika. Simmer for an additional 10•15 minutes, until vegetables are tender.

3. Season with salt and black pepper to taste. Serve the Lentil and Vegetable Soup warm, garnished with chopped parsley if desired.

Both of these lentil soup recipes are vegan and use ingredients that are easy to digest for those without a gallbladder, such as lentils, vegetables, and spices. The soups provide fiber, protein, and essential nutrients.

51. Vegan Pancakes with Fresh Berries

Ingredient:

- 1 cup all•purpose flour
- 1 tablespoon baking powder
- 1/4 teaspoon salt
- 1 cup unsweetened almond milk (or other non•dairy milk)
- 2 tablespoons maple syrup
- 1 tablespoon lemon juice
- 1 teaspoon vanilla extract
- 1 cup fresh berries (such as blueberries, raspberries, or sliced strawberries)

Instructions:

1. In a medium bowl, whisk together the flour, baking powder, and salt.

2. In a separate bowl, whisk together the almond milk, maple syrup, lemon juice, and vanilla extract.

3. Pour the wet ingredients into the dry ingredients and stir just until combined (do not overmix).

4. Heat a non•stick skillet or griddle over medium heat. Scoop about 1/4 cup of batter per pancake onto the hot surface.

5. Cook for 2•3 minutes per side, or until golden brown. Flip the pancakes gently with a spatula.

6. Serve the pancakes warm, topped with the fresh berries.

These vegan pancakes are a great option for those without a gallbladder, as they are free of dairy, eggs, and other ingredients that can be difficult to digest. The almond milk and lemon juice provide the necessary acidity and moisture without the need for eggs or butter. Enjoy these delicious and nutritious pancakes!

52. Tofu Scramble with Spinach

Ingredient:

• 1 block (14 oz) firm or extra•firm tofu, drained and crumbled
• 2 tablespoons olive oil
• 1 small onion, diced
• 3 cloves garlic, minced
• 1 cup fresh spinach, chopped
• 1 teaspoon ground turmeric
• 1 teaspoon ground cumin
• 1/2 teaspoon smoked paprika
• 1/4 teaspoon salt
• 1/4 teaspoon black pepper
• 2 tablespoons unsweetened almond milk (or other non•dairy milk)

Instructions:

1. Heat the olive oil in a large skillet over medium heat. Add the diced onion and sauté for 3•4 minutes until translucent.

2. Add the minced garlic and sauté for an additional minute until fragrant.

3. Crumble the tofu into the skillet and use a spatula to break it up into small pieces.

4. Stir in the turmeric, cumin, smoked paprika, salt, and black pepper. Mix well to coat the tofu.

5. Add the chopped spinach and the almond milk. Stir to combine and cook for 2•3 minutes, or until the spinach is wilted.

6. Taste and adjust seasonings as needed. Serve the tofu scramble warm.

This tofu scramble is a great source of plant•based protein and is easy to digest, making it a perfect gallbladder•friendly meal. The spinach adds extra nutrients and fiber. Enjoy this delicious and nutritious breakfast or brunch dish!

53. Oatmeal with Fresh Fruit

Ingredient:

• 1 cup rolled oats
• 2 cups unsweetened almond milk (or other non•dairy milk)
• 1 tablespoon maple syrup (or honey, if not vegan)
• 1/4 teaspoon ground cinnamon
• 1/8 teaspoon ground nutmeg
• 1 cup mixed fresh fruit (such as berries, sliced bananas, diced apples, etc.)

Instructions:

1. In a medium saucepan, combine the rolled oats and almond milk. Bring to a simmer over medium heat, stirring occasionally.

2. Once the oatmeal begins to thicken, about 5•7 minutes, reduce the heat to low and continue cooking for an additional 2•3 minutes, stirring frequently, until the oatmeal reaches your desired consistency.

3. Remove the oatmeal from the heat and stir in the maple syrup, cinnamon, and nutmeg.

4. Divide the oatmeal into serving bowls and top with the fresh mixed fruit.

5. Serve the oatmeal warm, with additional almond milk or maple syrup on the side if desired.

This vegan oatmeal dish is a great option for those without a gallbladder, as it is easy to digest and packed with fiber, vitamins, and minerals from the oats and fresh fruit. The almond milk provides a creamy texture without the use of dairy products. Feel free to adjust the fruit and spices to your personal taste preferences.

54. Chia Seed Pudding

Ingredient:

• 1/2 cup chia seeds
• 2 cups unsweetened almond milk (or other non•dairy milk)
• 2 tablespoons maple syrup (or honey, if not vegan)
• 1 teaspoon vanilla extract
• 1/4 teaspoon ground cinnamon
• 1 cup fresh berries (such as blueberries, raspberries, or sliced strawberries)

Instructions:

1. In a medium bowl, whisk together the chia seeds, almond milk, maple syrup, vanilla extract, and cinnamon until well combined.

2. Cover the bowl and refrigerate for at least 4 hours, or overnight, stirring occasionally, until the chia seeds have thickened the mixture into a pudding•like consistency.

3. When ready to serve, divide the chia seed pudding into individual serving bowls or glasses.

4. Top each serving with 1/4 cup of the fresh berries.

5. Serve chilled and enjoy!

This chia seed pudding is a great option for those without a gallbladder, as chia seeds are easy to digest and the almond milk provides a creamy texture without the use of dairy products. The fresh berries add a burst of natural sweetness and antioxidants.

You can also experiment with different flavor combinations, such as adding cocoa powder for a chocolate version, or using different types of fruit or nuts as toppings. The versatility of this recipe makes it a great healthy and satisfying snack or dessert.

55. Smoothie Bowl with Granola

Ingredient:

Smoothie:
• 1 cup frozen mixed berries (such as blueberries, raspberries, and strawberries)
• 1 banana, frozen
• 1 cup unsweetened almond milk (or other non•dairy milk)
• 2 tablespoons almond butter
• 1 tablespoon chia seeds
• 1 teaspoon vanilla extract

Granola Topping:
• 1 cup rolled oats
• 1/4 cup sliced almonds
• 2 tablespoons maple syrup
• 1 tablespoon coconut oil, melted
• 1/2 teaspoon ground cinnamon
• 1/4 teaspoon salt

Instructions:

1. Make the smoothie: In a high•speed blender, combine the frozen mixed berries, frozen banana, almond milk, almond butter, chia seeds, and vanilla extract. Blend until smooth and creamy.

2. Make the granola topping: Preheat the oven to 325°F (165°C). In a medium bowl, mix together the rolled oats, sliced almonds, maple syrup, melted coconut oil, cinnamon, and salt until well combined.

3. Spread the granola mixture onto a baking sheet lined with parchment paper. Bake for 15•20 minutes, stirring halfway, until the granola is golden brown and crispy.

4. Remove the granola from the oven and let it cool completely.

5. To assemble the smoothie bowl, pour the smoothie into a bowl and top with the cooled granola. You can also add additional fresh fruit, such as sliced bananas or berries, if desired.

This smoothie bowl is a great option for those without a gallbladder, as it is packed with fiber, healthy fats, and nutrients from the fruits, nuts, and seeds. The granola topping adds a satisfying crunch and extra texture. Enjoy this delicious and nutritious breakfast or snack!

56. Avocado Toast on Whole Grain Bread

Ingredient:

- 2 slices of whole grain bread
- 1 ripe avocado, mashed
- 1 tablespoon fresh lemon juice
- 1/4 teaspoon salt
- 1/8 teaspoon black pepper
- 1 tablespoon chopped fresh cilantro or parsley (optional)

Instructions:

1. Toast the whole grain bread slices until lightly golden brown.

2. In a small bowl, mash the avocado with a fork. Stir in the lemon juice, salt, and black pepper until well combined.

3. Spread the mashed avocado mixture evenly over the toasted bread slices.

4. If desired, sprinkle the chopped fresh cilantro or parsley over the top of the avocado toast.

5. Serve immediately and enjoy!

This avocado toast is a great option for those without a gallbladder, as it is easy to digest and packed with healthy fats, fiber, and nutrients. The whole grain bread provides complex carbohydrates, while the avocado is a great source of monounsaturated fats.

You can customize this recipe by adding other toppings, such as sliced tomatoes, radishes, or a drizzle of olive oil or balsamic glaze. This makes for a satisfying and nutritious breakfast, snack, or light meal.

Remember to choose ripe, creamy avocados for the best texture and flavor. Enjoy this delicious and gallbladder•friendly avocado toast!

57. Fruit Salad with Mint

Ingredient:

- 1 cup diced pineapple
- 1 cup diced mango
- 1 cup halved strawberries
- 1 cup blueberries
- 1 cup diced kiwi
- 2 tablespoons freshly chopped mint leaves
- 1 tablespoon lemon juice
- 1 tablespoon maple syrup (optional)

Instructions:

1. In a large bowl, combine the diced pineapple, mango, strawberries, blueberries, and kiwi.

2. Add the freshly chopped mint leaves and lemon juice. Gently toss to combine.

3. If desired, drizzle the maple syrup over the fruit salad and toss again to coat.

4. Cover the bowl and refrigerate the fruit salad for at least 30 minutes to allow the flavors to meld.

5. Serve the chilled fruit salad as a refreshing and healthy snack or side dish.

This fruit salad is a great option for those without a gallbladder, as it is easy to digest and packed with a variety of vitamins, minerals, and antioxidants from the different fruits. The mint adds a refreshing and aromatic touch, while the lemon juice helps to balance the sweetness.

You can adjust the fruit selection based on your preferences and what's in season. Other great options include diced apples, grapes, melon, or berries. The maple syrup is optional, as the fruit should provide enough natural sweetness.

Enjoy this vibrant and nutritious fruit salad as a light and refreshing snack or dessert.

58. Vegan Breakfast Burrito

Ingredient:

- 1 block (14 oz) firm or extra•firm tofu, crumbled
- 1 tablespoon olive oil
- 1 small onion, diced
- 1 red bell pepper, diced
- 2 cloves garlic, minced
- 1 teaspoon ground cumin
- 1 teaspoon chili powder
- 1/2 teaspoon smoked paprika
- 1/4 teaspoon salt
- 1/4 teaspoon black pepper
- 1/2 cup cooked black beans (or pinto beans)
- 4 whole wheat or gluten•free tortillas
- 1 avocado, sliced
- 1/2 cup shredded vegan cheese (optional)

Instructions:

1. In a large skillet, heat the olive oil over medium heat. Add the diced onion and bell pepper, and sauté for 5•7 minutes until softened.

2. Add the minced garlic and crumbled tofu to the skillet. Stir in the cumin, chili powder, smoked paprika, salt, and black pepper. Cook for 5•7 minutes, stirring occasionally, until the tofu is heated through and the flavors have blended.

3. Stir in the cooked black beans and heat through.

4. Warm the tortillas according to package instructions.

5. To assemble the burritos, place a portion of the tofu•bean mixture onto the center of each tortilla. Top with sliced avocado and shredded vegan cheese (if using).

6. Fold the bottom of the tortilla up over the filling, then fold in the sides and continue rolling up tightly to create a burrito. Serve the vegan breakfast burritos warm and enjoy!

This vegan breakfast burrito is a great option for those without a gallbladder, as it is easy to digest and packed with plant•based protein, fiber, and healthy fats. The combination of tofu, beans, and avocado provides a satisfying and nutritious meal.

Feel free to customize the fillings to your liking, such as adding sautéed mushrooms, spinach, or salsa. Enjoy this delicious and gallbladder•friendly breakfast burrito!

59. Buckwheat Pancakes

Ingredient:

• 1 cup buckwheat flour
• 1 tablespoon baking powder
• 1/4 teaspoon salt
• 1 cup unsweetened almond milk (or other non•dairy milk)
• 2 tablespoons maple syrup
• 1 tablespoon lemon juice
• 1 teaspoon vanilla extract

Toppings (optional):
• Fresh berries
• Sliced bananas
• Maple syrup
• Chopped nuts or seeds

Instructions:

1. In a medium bowl, whisk together the buckwheat flour, baking powder, and salt.

2. In a separate bowl, whisk together the almond milk, maple syrup, lemon juice, and vanilla extract.

3. Pour the wet ingredients into the dry ingredients and stir just until combined (do not overmix).

4. Heat a non•stick skillet or griddle over medium heat. Scoop about 1/4 cup of batter per pancake onto the hot surface.

5. Cook for 2•3 minutes per side, or until golden brown. Flip the pancakes gently with a spatula.

6. Serve the buckwheat pancakes warm, topped with your desired toppings such as fresh berries, sliced bananas, maple syrup, and/or chopped nuts or seeds.

These vegan buckwheat pancakes are a great option for those without a gallbladder, as buckwheat is easy to digest and gluten•free. The almond milk and lemon juice provide the necessary acidity and moisture without the need for eggs or dairy.

Buckwheat is a nutrient•dense grain that is high in fiber, protein, and antioxidants. It's a great alternative to traditional wheat•based pancakes, making this a healthy and satisfying breakfast or brunch option.

60. Coconut Yogurt with Nuts and Seeds

Ingredient:

- 1 cup unsweetened coconut yogurt
- 2 tablespoons chopped raw almonds
- 2 tablespoons chopped raw walnuts
- 1 tablespoon chia seeds
- 1 tablespoon hemp seeds
- 1 tablespoon unsweetened shredded coconut
- 1 tablespoon maple syrup (optional)

Instructions:

1. In a medium bowl, scoop the coconut yogurt.

2. Sprinkle the chopped almonds, walnuts, chia seeds, and hemp seeds over the top of the yogurt.

3. Garnish with the unsweetened shredded coconut.

4. If desired, drizzle the maple syrup over the top of the yogurt and toppings.

5. Serve chilled and enjoy!

This coconut yogurt with nuts and seeds is a great option for those without a gallbladder, as it is easy to digest and packed with healthy fats, protein, and fiber.

The coconut yogurt provides a creamy and probiotic•rich base, while the nuts and seeds add a satisfying crunch and additional nutrients. The chia and hemp seeds are great sources of omega•3 fatty acids, which can be beneficial for gallbladder health.

You can adjust the amounts and types of nuts and seeds based on your preferences. Other great options include pecans, cashews, pumpkin seeds, or sunflower seeds.

The maple syrup is optional, as the natural sweetness of the coconut yogurt and the crunch of the nuts and seeds should provide enough flavor. Enjoy this delicious and nutritious breakfast or snack!

61. Fruit Sorbet

Ingredient:

- 2 cups frozen fruit (such as mango, pineapple, or mixed berries)
- 1/4 cup unsweetened almond milk (or other non•dairy milk)
- 1 tablespoon maple syrup (optional)
- 1 tablespoon fresh lemon or lime juice

Instructions:

1. In a high•speed blender or food processor, combine the frozen fruit, almond milk, maple syrup (if using), and lemon or lime juice.

2. Blend or process the mixture until it reaches a smooth, sorbet•like consistency, scraping down the sides as needed.

3. Taste and adjust sweetness or acidity as desired, adding more maple syrup or lemon/lime juice if needed.

4. Serve the fruit sorbet immediately, or transfer it to an airtight container and freeze for 1•2 hours, stirring occasionally, until it reaches your desired frozen consistency.

5. Scoop the sorbet into bowls or glasses and enjoy!

This fruit sorbet is a great option for those without a gallbladder, as it is easy to digest and packed with vitamins, minerals, and antioxidants from the fresh fruit. The almond milk provides a creamy texture without the use of dairy products.

You can use a variety of frozen fruits to create different flavors, such as mango, pineapple, strawberry, or mixed berries. The maple syrup is optional, as the natural sweetness of the fruit should be enough.

This sorbet is a refreshing and healthy dessert or palate cleanser, perfect for hot summer days or as a light and satisfying snack. Enjoy this delicious and gallbladder•friendly fruit sorbet!

62. Dark Chocolate Covered Strawberries

Ingredient:

• 1 cup fresh strawberries, washed and dried thoroughly
• 4 oz dark chocolate (at least 70% cacao), chopped
• 1 tablespoon coconut oil

Instructions:

1. Line a baking sheet or plate with parchment paper.

2. In a double boiler or a heatproof bowl set over a saucepan of simmering water, melt the chopped dark chocolate and coconut oil, stirring occasionally until smooth.

3. Carefully dip each strawberry into the melted chocolate, coating it about three•quarters of the way up. Gently tap off any excess chocolate.

4. Place the chocolate•dipped strawberries on the prepared baking sheet or plate.

5. Refrigerate the chocolate•covered strawberries for at least 30 minutes, or until the chocolate has hardened.

6. Serve the dark chocolate covered strawberries chilled and enjoy!

These dark chocolate covered strawberries are a great option for those without a gallbladder, as they are easy to digest and provide a satisfying sweet treat.

The dark chocolate is rich in antioxidants and the strawberries are a good source of fiber, vitamins, and minerals. The coconut oil helps to create a smooth, glossy coating on the strawberries.

You can experiment with different types of dark chocolate or even try using vegan chocolate chips or bars. The key is to use a high•quality, high•cacao content chocolate for the best flavor and health benefits.

Enjoy these delicious and nutritious dark chocolate covered strawberries as a healthy dessert or snack option.

63. Vegan Chocolate Mousse

Ingredient:

• 1 (15 oz) can full•fat coconut milk, chilled overnight
• 1/2 cup unsweetened cocoa powder
• 1/4 cup maple syrup
• 1 teaspoon vanilla extract
• 1/4 teaspoon sea salt

Instructions:

1. Chill a medium•sized mixing bowl in the refrigerator for at least 30 minutes.

2. Carefully open the chilled can of coconut milk without shaking it. Scoop out the thick, creamy coconut solids, leaving the watery coconut milk behind (save the coconut milk for another use).

3. Add the coconut solids to the chilled mixing bowl. Using a hand mixer or stand mixer fitted with the whisk attachment, whip the coconut solids on high speed for 2•3 minutes until light and fluffy.

4. Add the cocoa powder, maple syrup, vanilla extract, and sea salt to the whipped coconut cream. Beat on high speed for an additional 2•3 minutes until the mixture is smooth and creamy.

5. Divide the chocolate mousse into individual serving dishes or ramekins.

6. Refrigerate the vegan chocolate mousse for at least 2 hours, or until set, before serving.

This vegan chocolate mousse is a delightful and indulgent dessert that is also gentle on the gallbladder. The rich, creamy texture comes from the coconut milk, while the cocoa powder and maple syrup provide the chocolate flavor.

You can top the mousse with fresh berries, chopped nuts, or a dusting of cocoa powder for an extra special touch. This recipe is also easily scalable, so you can make a larger batch for a crowd.

Enjoy this decadent and gallbladder•friendly vegan chocolate mousse!

64. Chia Seed Fruit Pudding

Ingredient:

• 1 cup unsweetened almond milk (or milk of your choice)
• 3 tablespoons chia seeds
• 1 cup diced fresh fruit (such as strawberries, blueberries, mango, etc.)
• 1•2 tablespoons honey or maple syrup (optional)
• 1/2 teaspoon vanilla extract (optional)

Instructions:

1. In a medium bowl, whisk together the almond milk and chia seeds until well combined.

2. Cover the bowl and refrigerate for at least 2 hours, or up to overnight, stirring occasionally, until the chia seeds have thickened the mixture into a pudding•like consistency.

3. Once the chia pudding has set, stir in the diced fruit.

4. If desired, drizzle in the honey or maple syrup and vanilla extract, and stir to combine.

5. Serve the chia seed fruit pudding chilled, either as is or with additional toppings such as:
   • Toasted coconut flakes
   • Chopped nuts
   • Fresh mint leaves
   • A sprinkle of cinnamon

Tips:
• Use a variety of fresh, seasonal fruits for different flavors and colors.
• Adjust the amount of honey or maple syrup to your desired sweetness level.
• Prepare the chia pudding base in advance for a quick and easy breakfast or snack.
• This recipe can be easily doubled or tripled to make a larger batch.

Enjoy your healthy and delicious chia seed fruit pudding!

65. Coconut Macaroons

Ingredient:

• 3 large egg whites
• 1/2 cup granulated sugar
• 1/4 teaspoon salt
• 2 1/2 cups sweetened shredded coconut

Instructions:

1. Preheat the oven to 325°F (165°C). Line a baking sheet with parchment paper.

2. In a medium bowl, beat the egg whites with an electric mixer until they are foamy. Gradually add the sugar and salt, beating until the mixture forms stiff, glossy peaks.

3. Gently fold in the shredded coconut until well combined.

4. Scoop rounded tablespoons of the coconut mixture onto the prepared baking sheet, spacing them about 1 inch apart.

5. Bake for 18•20 minutes, until the macaroons are lightly golden brown on the edges.

6. Remove the baking sheet from the oven and let the macaroons cool on the sheet for 5 minutes before transferring them to a wire rack to cool completely.

Tips:
• For chunkier macaroons, use unsweetened shredded coconut instead of sweetened.
• You can dip the bottoms of the cooled macaroons in melted chocolate for an extra treat.
• Store the macaroons in an airtight container at room temperature for up to 1 week.

Enjoy your homemade coconut macaroons!

66. Vegan Lemon Bars

Ingredient:

- 1 1/2 cups all•purpose flour
- 1/2 cup powdered sugar
- 1/2 cup vegan butter, chilled and cubed

Filling Ingredients:

- 1 cup freshly squeezed lemon juice (about 4•5 lemons)
- 1 cup granulated sugar
- 1/2 cup aquafaba (liquid from a can of chickpeas)
- 1/4 cup all•purpose flour
- 1/4 teaspoon salt

Instructions:

For the Crust:

1. Preheat the oven to 350°F (175°C). Grease an 8x8 inch baking pan.
2. In a food processor, pulse the flour, powdered sugar, and vegan butter until the mixture resembles coarse crumbs.
3. Press the crust mixture evenly into the prepared baking pan.
4. Bake for 15•18 minutes, until lightly golden. Allow to cool completely.

For the Filling:

1. In a medium saucepan, whisk together the lemon juice, granulated sugar, aquafaba, flour, and salt.

2. Cook over medium heat, stirring constantly, until the mixture thickens and bubbles, about 5•7 minutes.

3. Pour the hot lemon filling over the cooled crust.

4. Bake for an additional 18•22 minutes, until the filling is set.

5. Allow the bars to cool completely, then refrigerate for at least 2 hours before cutting and serving. Dust with powdered sugar before serving, if desired.

Tips:

- Use fresh, juicy lemons for the best flavor.
- Aquafaba helps create a creamy, custard•like filling.
- Chill the bars thoroughly before cutting for clean, neat slices.
- Store leftovers in the refrigerator for up to 5 days.

67. Almond Butter Cookies

Ingredient:

- 1 cup creamy almond butter
- 1 cup granulated sugar
- 1 large egg
- 1 teaspoon baking soda
- 1/4 teaspoon salt

Instructions:

1. Preheat your oven to 350°F (175°C). Line a baking sheet with parchment paper.

2. In a medium bowl, combine the almond butter, sugar, egg, baking soda, and salt. Mix until the ingredients are well incorporated and a smooth dough forms.

3. Scoop rounded tablespoons of the dough and place them about 2 inches apart on the prepared baking sheet.

4. Using a fork, gently press down on each cookie to create a criss•cross pattern on the top.

5. Bake the cookies for 8•10 minutes, or until the edges are lightly golden brown.

6. Remove the cookies from the oven and let them cool on the baking sheet for 5 minutes before transferring them to a wire rack to cool completely.

Tips:
- For a chunkier texture, use crunchy almond butter instead of creamy.
- You can add 1/2 cup of chopped toasted almonds or chocolate chips to the dough for extra flavor.
- Store the cooled cookies in an airtight container at room temperature for up to 1 week.

Enjoy your delicious and easy•to•make almond butter cookies!

68. Pumpkin Pie (using vegan crust)

Ingredient:

- 1 1/4 cups all•purpose flour
- 1/2 teaspoon salt
- 1/2 cup cold vegan butter, cubed
- 3•4 tablespoons ice water

Filling Ingredients:
- 1 (15 oz) can pumpkin puree

- 1 cup unsweetened almond milk (or other non•dairy milk)
- 3/4 cup brown sugar
- 2 teaspoons ground cinnamon
- 1 teaspoon ground ginger
- 1/2 teaspoon ground nutmeg
- 1/4 teaspoon ground cloves
- 1/4 teaspoon salt
- 1 tablespoon cornstarch

Instructions:

For the Crust:
1. In a food processor, pulse the flour and salt together. Add the cold vegan butter and pulse until the mixture resembles coarse crumbs.

2. Add the ice water 1 tablespoon at a time, pulsing after each addition, until the dough just begins to hold together.

3. Turn the dough out onto a lightly floured surface and shape into a disc. Wrap in plastic wrap and refrigerate for at least 30 minutes.

4. Roll out the dough into a 12•inch circle and transfer to a 9•inch pie plate. Crimp the edges as desired.

For the Filling:
1. Preheat the oven to 375°F (190°C).

2. In a large bowl, whisk together the pumpkin puree, almond milk, brown sugar, cinnamon, ginger, nutmeg, cloves, and salt until well combined.

3. Whisk in the cornstarch until no lumps remain.

4. Pour the filling into the prepared pie crust.

5. Bake for 45•55 minutes, or until the center is almost set. The pie should still have a slight jiggle in the center. Allow the pie to cool completely on a wire rack before slicing and serving.

69. Banana Ice Cream

Ingredient:

- 3•4 ripe bananas, peeled and frozen
- 2•3 tablespoons non•dairy milk (such as almond, coconut, or oat milk)
- 1 teaspoon vanilla extract (optional)
- Pinch of salt (optional)

Instructions:

1. Place the frozen banana slices in a high•powered blender or food processor.

2. Add 2•3 tablespoons of non•dairy milk, starting with the smaller amount. The amount of milk needed will depend on the consistency you prefer.

3. Blend or process the bananas and milk until smooth and creamy, scraping down the sides as needed. The mixture should have a soft, ice cream•like texture.

4. If desired, add 1 teaspoon of vanilla extract and a pinch of salt. Blend again briefly to incorporate.

5. Serve the banana ice cream immediately for a soft•serve consistency, or transfer it to an airtight container and freeze for 2•3 hours for a firmer, scoopable texture.

Tips:
- Ripe, spotty bananas work best for this recipe as they are sweeter and creamier.
- Freeze the bananas in a single layer on a baking sheet before blending for best results.
- For a thicker, creamier ice cream, use less non•dairy milk.
- Add mix•ins like peanut butter, cocoa powder, or chopped nuts for extra flavor.
- Scoop the banana ice cream into bowls or cones and enjoy immediately for a refreshing treat.

This simple, 3•ingredient banana ice cream is a healthy, dairy•free alternative to traditional ice cream. Enjoy!

70. Stuffed Dates with Almond Butter

Ingredient:

- 12 Medjool dates, pitted
- 1/4 cup creamy almond butter
- 2 tablespoons chopped roasted almonds (optional)

Instructions:

1. Slice each date lengthwise, being careful not to cut all the way through. You want to create a pocket for the almond butter.

2. Spoon about 1·2 teaspoons of almond butter into the pocket of each date.

3. If desired, sprinkle the chopped roasted almonds over the top of the stuffed dates.

4. Arrange the stuffed dates on a serving plate or platter.

5. Refrigerate the stuffed dates for at least 30 minutes before serving to allow the almond butter to firm up slightly.

6. Serve the chilled stuffed dates as a healthy and satisfying snack.

These stuffed dates with almond butter are a great option for those without a gallbladder, as they are easy to digest and provide a good source of healthy fats, fiber, and protein.

The Medjool dates are naturally sweet and chewy, while the creamy almond butter adds a rich and nutty flavor. The optional chopped almonds provide a nice crunch and additional texture.

You can experiment with different nut butters, such as peanut butter or cashew butter, if desired. Just be sure to choose a natural, unsweetened variety for the best nutritional profile.

Enjoy these delicious and nutritious stuffed dates as a quick and satisfying snack or small dessert. They're perfect for satisfying sweet cravings in a healthy way.

71. Fresh Fruit Smoothie

Ingredient:

- 1 cup frozen mixed berries (such as blueberries, raspberries, and strawberries)
- 1 banana, frozen
- 1 cup unsweetened almond milk
- 1 tablespoon almond butter
- 1 tablespoon chia seeds
- 1 teaspoon vanilla extract

Instructions:

1. In a high•speed blender, combine the frozen mixed berries, frozen banana, almond milk, almond butter, chia seeds, and vanilla extract.

2. Blend the ingredients on high speed until the smoothie is smooth and creamy, about 1•2 minutes.

3. Taste the smoothie and adjust any ingredients as needed, such as adding more almond milk for a thinner consistency or more chia seeds for extra thickness.

4. Pour the fresh fruit smoothie into a glass and enjoy immediately.

This fresh fruit smoothie is a great option for those without a gallbladder, as it is easy to digest and packed with nutrients. The frozen fruit provides a naturally sweet and creamy base, while the almond milk and almond butter add healthy fats and creaminess without the use of dairy products.

The chia seeds are a great source of fiber, protein, and omega•3 fatty acids, which can be beneficial for gallbladder health.

You can experiment with different fruit combinations, such as mango, pineapple, or kiwi, to create your own unique flavor profiles. You can also add other nutrient•dense ingredients like spinach, kale, or ground flaxseeds.

Enjoy this refreshing and nutritious fresh fruit smoothie as a healthy snack or light meal.

72. Green Tea

Ingredient:

• 1 teaspoon loose•leaf green tea or 1 green tea bag
• 1 cup freshly boiled water

Instructions:

1. Bring fresh, cold water to a boil in a kettle or on the stove. The water should reach a temperature of 160•180°F (71•82°C), which is just below a full rolling boil.

2. Place the green tea leaves or tea bag in a teapot or mug.

3. Pour the hot water over the tea leaves/bag.

4. Allow the tea to steep for 2•3 minutes. Do not over•steep, as this can make the tea taste bitter.

5. Strain the tea leaves or remove the tea bag.

6. Pour the brewed green tea into your cup and enjoy!

Tips:
• Use fresh, high•quality green tea leaves or bags for best flavor.
• Adjust steeping time to your taste preference • less time for a lighter flavor, longer for a stronger brew.
• You can add a squeeze of lemon, a drizzle of honey, or a sprig of mint to complement the green tea flavor.
• Drink the green tea while it's hot for maximum health benefits and flavor.

Enjoy your freshly brewed green tea!

73. Herbal Tea

Ingredient:

• 1 teaspoon dried herbal tea blend (such as chamomile, peppermint, lemon balm, etc.)
• 1 cup freshly boiled water

Instructions:

1. Bring fresh, cold water to a boil in a kettle or on the stove.

2. Place the dried herbal tea blend in a teapot or mug.

3. Pour the hot water over the herbs and let the tea steep for 5•7 minutes.

4. Strain the tea leaves or remove the tea bag, if using.

5. Pour the brewed herbal tea into your cup and enjoy!

Herbal Tea Blend Ideas:
• Chamomile, lavender, and lemon balm (for relaxation)
• Peppermint, ginger, and lemon (for digestion)
• Hibiscus, rosehip, and cinnamon (for antioxidants)
• Echinacea, elderberry, and ginger (for immune support)

Tips:
• Use 1•2 teaspoons of dried herbs per cup of water, adjusting to your taste preference.

• Steep the tea for 5•7 minutes to extract the maximum flavor and health benefits.

• You can add a touch of honey, lemon, or a cinnamon stick to enhance the flavor.

• Store any leftover dried herbal tea blend in an airtight container in a cool, dark place.

Enjoy your soothing and healthy homemade herbal tea!

74. Iced Mint Tea

Ingredient:

- 6 cups water
- 1/2 cup fresh mint leaves, lightly packed
- 2 tablespoons honey (or to taste)
- Lemon slices (optional)
- Ice cubes

Instructions:

1. In a medium saucepan, bring the water to a boil over high heat.

2. Remove the pan from the heat and add the fresh mint leaves. Allow the mint to steep for 5•7 minutes.

3. Strain the mint tea through a fine•mesh sieve or cheesecloth, discarding the used mint leaves.

4. Stir in the honey until it's fully dissolved. Taste and add more honey if desired.

5. Allow the mint tea to cool to room temperature.

6. Fill a pitcher or glasses with ice cubes. Pour the cooled mint tea over the ice.

7. Garnish with fresh lemon slices, if desired.

Tips:
- Use a variety of fresh mint, such as spearmint or peppermint, for different flavor profiles.
- For a stronger mint flavor, you can bruise or lightly crush the mint leaves before steeping.
- Adjust the amount of honey to your personal taste preferences.
- Serve the iced mint tea immediately for the best flavor and texture.
- Store any leftover tea in the refrigerator for up to 4 days.

Enjoy your refreshing and flavorful iced mint tea!

75. Almond Milk Latte

Ingredient:

• 1 cup unsweetened almond milk
• 1•2 shots of espresso or strong brewed coffee
• 1 teaspoon maple syrup (optional)
• Ground cinnamon for dusting (optional)

Instructions:

1. In a small saucepan, heat the almond milk over medium heat, stirring occasionally, until steaming hot but not boiling.

2. Using a milk frother or a small whisk, vigorously froth the hot almond milk until it becomes light and creamy.

3. Pour the frothed almond milk into a mug or glass.

4. Carefully pour the espresso or strong brewed coffee over the frothed almond milk.

5. If desired, stir in the maple syrup to sweeten the latte.

6. Dust the top of the latte with a light sprinkle of ground cinnamon.

7. Serve the almond milk latte immediately while hot and enjoy!

This almond milk latte is a great option for those without a gallbladder, as almond milk is easy to digest and doesn't contain any dairy products. The espresso or coffee provides a caffeine boost, while the maple syrup (if used) adds a touch of natural sweetness.

You can adjust the ratio of almond milk to coffee/espresso to suit your personal taste preferences. For a creamier latte, use more almond milk, and for a stronger coffee flavor, use more espresso or coffee.

Feel free to experiment with different flavor variations, such as adding a dash of vanilla extract or using different types of sweeteners like honey or agave nectar.

Enjoy this delicious and gallbladder•friendly almond milk latte as a comforting and satisfying beverage.

76. Coconut Water

Ingredient:

• 1 young green coconut

Instructions:

1. Carefully pierce the coconut with a sharp knife or screwdriver to create a hole. Drain the coconut water into a glass or container.

2. Using a cleaver or heavy knife, carefully crack open the coconut by striking it along the equator until it splits in half.

3. Use a spoon to scoop out the soft, jelly•like coconut meat from the shell.

4. Optionally, you can blend or process the coconut meat with the coconut water to create a creamy coconut beverage.

Tips:

• Look for young, green coconuts that have a thin, soft husk and plenty of liquid inside.

• Avoid coconuts that feel heavy and have a sloshing sound, as they may be old and have less water.

• Drink the coconut water immediately for maximum freshness and nutrient retention.

• You can add a squeeze of lime juice or a pinch of salt to the coconut water for extra flavor.

• Store any leftover coconut water in an airtight container in the refrigerator for up to 3•4 days.

• The coconut meat can be used in various recipes, such as curries, smoothies, or desserts.

Enjoy the refreshing and hydrating benefits of fresh, homemade coconut water!

77. Vegetable Juice

Ingredient:

- 2 carrots, peeled and chopped
- 1 cucumber, peeled and chopped
- 1 celery stalk, chopped
- 1 cup spinach or kale, packed
- 1 apple, cored and chopped
- 1·inch piece of ginger, peeled
- 1 lemon, juiced
- 1 cup water (optional)

Instructions:

1. Wash all the vegetables and fruits thoroughly.

2. Add the chopped carrots, cucumber, celery, spinach/kale, apple, and ginger to a high·powered blender or juicer.

3. If using a blender, add the 1 cup of water to help the blending process. If using a juicer, skip the water.

4. Blend or juice the ingredients until you achieve a smooth, liquid consistency.

5. Stir in the lemon juice.

6. Pour the vegetable juice into glasses and serve immediately.

Tips:
• Adjust the amounts of each ingredient to suit your taste preferences.

• You can use a variety of vegetables and fruits, such as beets, tomatoes, parsley, or pineapple.

• For a creamier texture, you can add a small avocado to the blend.

• Drink the juice right away for maximum nutrient retention.

• Store any leftover juice in an airtight container in the refrigerator for up to 3 days.

Enjoy your refreshing and nutritious homemade vegetable juice!

78. Fresh Lemonade

Ingredient:

• 6 lemons, juiced (about 1 cup of lemon juice)
• 3/4 cup granulated sugar
• 4 cups cold water
• Ice cubes
• Lemon slices for garnish (optional)

Instructions:

1. In a large pitcher, stir together the lemon juice and granulated sugar until the sugar is fully dissolved.

2. Add the cold water and stir to combine.

3. Taste the lemonade and adjust the sweetness by adding more sugar if desired.

4. Fill glasses with ice cubes and pour the fresh lemonade over the ice.

5. Garnish each glass with a lemon slice, if desired.

Tips:

• Use fresh, ripe lemons for the best flavor. You can use a combination of lemon varieties for added complexity.

• Adjust the sugar amount to your personal taste preferences. Start with less sugar and add more if you want a sweeter lemonade.

• For a fizzy lemonade, replace some of the water with sparkling water or club soda.

• Add fresh mint leaves, sliced strawberries, or other fruit to the pitcher for a flavored lemonade.

• Refrigerate any leftover lemonade in an airtight container for up to 5 days.

Enjoy your refreshing homemade lemonade!

79. Sparkling Water with Lemon

Ingredient:

• 4 cups chilled sparkling water
• 1 lemon, sliced
• Ice cubes (optional)

Instructions:

1. Fill a pitcher or large glass with the chilled sparkling water.

2. Add the lemon slices to the sparkling water.

3. Stir gently to combine.

4. Pour the sparkling water with lemon over ice cubes in glasses, if desired.

Tips:

• Use freshly squeezed lemon juice instead of lemon slices for a more intense lemon flavor.

• Try using different citrus fruits, such as lime, orange, or grapefruit, for variety.

• Add a few mint leaves or a splash of fruit juice (such as cranberry or pomegranate) for extra flavor.

• Experiment with different types of sparkling water, such as plain, flavored, or mineral water.

• Serve the sparkling water with lemon immediately for maximum freshness and fizz.

• Store any leftover sparkling water in the refrigerator for up to 3 days.

This refreshing sparkling water with lemon is a great alternative to sugary sodas or juices. It's hydrating, low in calories, and easy to customize to your taste preferences.

Enjoy your homemade sparkling water with lemon!

80. Homemade Nut Milk

Ingredient:

• 1 cup raw, unsalted nuts (such as almonds, cashews, or a mix)
• 4 cups filtered water
• Pinch of salt (optional)
• Sweetener (such as maple syrup, honey, or dates) to taste (optional)

Instructions:

1. Soak the nuts in water for 4•8 hours, or overnight, in the refrigerator. This helps soften the nuts and makes them easier to blend.

2. Drain and rinse the soaked nuts.

3. Add the soaked nuts, 4 cups of fresh filtered water, and a pinch of salt (if using) to a high•powered blender.

4. Blend on high speed for 1•2 minutes, until the mixture is smooth and creamy.

5. Strain the nut milk through a nut milk bag, cheesecloth, or fine•mesh sieve, pressing on the solids to extract as much liquid as possible.

6. Discard the nut pulp or save it for other uses, such as baking or making nut butter.

7. If desired, stir in a sweetener (such as maple syrup, honey, or a few pitted dates) to taste.

8. Store the homemade nut milk in an airtight container in the refrigerator for up to 4•5 days.

Tips:
• Experiment with different types of nuts to find your favorite flavor.

• For a creamier texture, use fewer nuts or add a small amount of coconut oil or avocado.

• Adjust the sweetness to your preference or leave it unsweetened.

• Use the nut pulp in baked goods, smoothies, or to make nut butter. Shake or stir the nut milk before each use, as it may separate during storage.

81. Mixed Nuts

Ingredient:

• 1 cup raw, unsalted mixed nuts (such as almonds, cashews, pecans, walnuts, hazelnuts, etc.)
• 1 tablespoon olive oil or melted coconut oil (optional)
• 1 teaspoon sea salt or Himalayan salt (optional)
• 1/2 teaspoon ground cumin, chili powder, or other spices (optional)

Instructions:

1. Preheat your oven to 325°F (165°C).

2. If using oil, toss the mixed nuts with the oil in a medium bowl until they are lightly coated.

3. Spread the nuts in a single layer on a baking sheet.

4. If using salt and/or spices, sprinkle them evenly over the nuts.

5. Bake the nuts for 8•12 minutes, stirring halfway, until they are lightly toasted and fragrant.

6. Remove the nuts from the oven and let them cool completely on the baking sheet.

7. Once cooled, transfer the mixed nuts to an airtight container for storage.

Tips:

• Use a combination of your favorite raw, unsalted nuts for the best flavor and texture.

• Adjust the baking time as needed, keeping a close eye on the nuts to prevent burning.

• For flavored nuts, try using different spice blends, such as cajun seasoning, curry powder, or rosemary and garlic.

• Store the mixed nuts in an airtight container at room temperature for up to 2 weeks.

• You can also freeze the nuts for longer•term storage, up to 6 months. Serve the mixed nuts as a snack, add them to salads, or use them in baking recipes.

82. Rice Cakes with Nut Butter

Ingredient:

• 2•3 whole grain rice cakes
• 2•3 tablespoons of your favorite nut butter (such as peanut, almond, or cashew butter)
• Sliced fruit (such as banana, apple, or berries) (optional)
• Honey or maple syrup (optional)
• Cinnamon (optional)

Instructions:

1. Spread the nut butter evenly over the rice cakes.

2. Top the nut butter with sliced fruit, if desired.

3. Drizzle a small amount of honey or maple syrup over the fruit, if desired.

4. Sprinkle a pinch of cinnamon over the top, if desired.

That's it! Your rice cakes with nut butter are ready to enjoy.

Tips:

• Use a variety of nut butters to change up the flavor profile.
• Try different fruit combinations, such as sliced strawberries and bananas or apple and cinnamon.
• For extra protein, add a sprinkle of chopped nuts or seeds on top.
• Toast the rice cakes lightly before assembling for a crunchier texture.
• Store any leftover rice cakes with nut butter in an airtight container in the refrigerator for up to 3 days.

This simple, nutritious snack is a great way to satisfy your hunger and provide a boost of healthy fats, protein, and carbohydrates. Enjoy!

83. Popcorn (air•popped)

Ingredient:

• 1/2 cup unpopped popcorn kernels
• 1•2 tablespoons olive oil or avocado oil (optional)
• Sea salt or other seasonings (optional)

Instructions:

1. If using an air popper:
   • Plug in the air popper and place a large bowl underneath the chute.
   • Add the 1/2 cup of unpopped kernels to the air popper and turn it on.
   • Allow the popcorn to pop, stopping once the popping slows to 2•3 seconds between pops.

2. If popping on the stovetop:
   • In a large, heavy•bottomed pot with a tight•fitting lid, heat the 1•2 tablespoons of oil over medium•high heat.
   • Once the oil is hot, add the 1/2 cup of unpopped kernels in a single layer.
   • Cover the pot with the lid and keep the pot moving by shaking or swirling it to prevent burning.
   • Once the popping slows to 2•3 seconds between pops, remove the pot from the heat.

3. Transfer the freshly popped popcorn to a large bowl.

4. If desired, season the popcorn with sea salt or other seasonings, such as:
   • Garlic powder
   • Onion powder
   • Nutritional yeast
   • Chili powder
   • Dried herbs

Tips:

• Avoid using butter or other dairy products, as they can be difficult to digest for those without a gallbladder.
• Opt for healthy oils like olive oil or avocado oil, or skip the oil altogether for a lower•fat option.
• Experiment with different seasoning blends to find your favorite flavor combinations.
• Store any leftover popcorn in an airtight container at room temperature for up to 3 days.

84. Fruit Kabobs

Ingredient:

• Assorted fresh fruits (such as strawberries, pineapple, grapes, melon, kiwi, etc.)
• Wooden or metal skewers

Instructions:

1. Wash and prepare the fruits:
   • Cut larger fruits, like pineapple or melon, into bite•sized cubes or chunks.
   • Leave smaller fruits, like grapes or berries, whole.

2. Thread the prepared fruit onto the skewers, alternating colors and shapes for a visually appealing presentation.

3. Arrange the fruit kabobs on a serving platter or tray.

4. Optionally, you can serve the fruit kabobs with a dipping sauce, such as:
   • Honey•yogurt dip
   • Chocolate fondue
   • Caramel sauce
   • Whipped cream

Tips:

• Choose a variety of fruits with different colors, textures, and flavors for a more interesting kabob.

• Cut the fruits into similar•sized pieces to ensure even cooking and easy threading.

• Soak wooden skewers in water for 30 minutes before using to prevent them from burning.

• Refrigerate the prepared fruit kabobs until ready to serve for maximum freshness.

• Serve the fruit kabobs chilled or at room temperature.

• Customize the kabobs with additional toppings, such as toasted coconut, chopped nuts, or a drizzle of honey.

Enjoy these colorful and healthy fruit kabobs as a refreshing snack or dessert!

85. Roasted Chickpeas

Ingredient:

• 1 (15 oz) can chickpeas (garbanzo beans), drained and rinsed
• 1 tablespoon olive oil
• 1 teaspoon ground cumin
• 1 teaspoon paprika
• 1/2 teaspoon garlic powder
• 1/4 teaspoon salt
• 1/4 teaspoon black pepper

Instructions:

1. Preheat your oven to 400°F (200°C). Line a baking sheet with parchment paper.

2. Pat the drained and rinsed chickpeas dry with a paper towel or clean kitchen towel. This will help them get crispy in the oven.

3. In a medium bowl, toss the chickpeas with the olive oil, cumin, paprika, garlic powder, salt, and black pepper until the chickpeas are evenly coated.

4. Spread the seasoned chickpeas in a single layer on the prepared baking sheet.

5. Roast the chickpeas for 20•25 minutes, stirring halfway, until they are crispy and golden brown.

6. Remove the roasted chickpeas from the oven and let them cool for a few minutes before serving.

Tips:

• For extra crispiness, you can pat the chickpeas even drier before tossing them with the oil and spices.
• Experiment with different spice blends, such as chili powder, curry powder, or cajun seasoning.
• Roast the chickpeas at a higher temperature (425°F/220°C) for a crunchier texture.
• Toss the roasted chickpeas with a drizzle of honey or maple syrup for a sweet and savory snack.
• Store the roasted chickpeas in an airtight container at room temperature for up to 1 week.

86. Raw Veggie Sticks with Hummus

Ingredient:

Veggie Sticks:
• 1 medium carrot, peeled and cut into sticks
• 1 celery stalk, cut into sticks
• 1 cucumber, peeled and cut into sticks
• 1 red bell pepper, cut into strips
• 1 yellow bell pepper, cut into strips

Gallbladder•Friendly Hummus:
• 1 (15 oz) can chickpeas, drained and rinsed
• 1/4 cup tahini (sesame seed paste)
• 2 tablespoons olive oil
• 2 tablespoons lemon juice
• 1 garlic clove, minced
• 1/4 teaspoon ground cumin
• 1/4 teaspoon salt
• 2•3 tablespoons water, as needed

Instructions:

For the Hummus:
1. In a food processor or high•powered blender, combine the chickpeas, tahini, olive oil, lemon juice, garlic, cumin, and salt.
2. Blend the mixture, adding 2•3 tablespoons of water as needed, until smooth and creamy.
3. Taste and adjust seasoning as desired.

For the Veggie Sticks:
1. Wash and prepare the vegetables, cutting them into long, thin sticks.

To Serve:
1. Arrange the veggie sticks on a platter or plate.
2. Serve the homemade hummus alongside the veggie sticks for dipping.

Tips:
• Avoid using butter or dairy•based dips, as they can be difficult to digest for those without a gallbladder.
• Opt for healthy fats like olive oil and tahini in the hummus.
• You can also include other raw veggies, such as broccoli florets, cherry tomatoes, or snow pea pods.
• Store any leftover hummus in an airtight container in the refrigerator for up to 5 days.

87. Whole Grain Crackers with Salsa

Ingredient:

• 1 cup whole wheat flour (or gluten•free flour blend)
• 1/2 cup rolled oats
• 1/4 cup ground flaxseed
• 1/2 teaspoon salt
• 2•3 tablespoons olive oil or avocado oil
• 4•6 tablespoons water

Salsa Ingredients:
• 2 medium tomatoes, diced
• 1/2 red onion, finely chopped
• 1 jalapeño, seeded and finely chopped (optional)
• 1/4 cup chopped fresh cilantro
• 2 tablespoons lime juice
• 1/2 teaspoon salt

Instructions:
For the Crackers:
1. Preheat the oven to 350°F (175°C). Line a baking sheet with parchment paper.
2. In a medium bowl, mix together the whole wheat flour, rolled oats, ground flaxseed, and salt.
3. Add the olive oil and 4 tablespoons of water, and mix until a dough forms. Add more water as needed if the dough is too dry.
4. Roll the dough out between two sheets of parchment paper to about 1/8•inch thickness.
5. Transfer the dough (still between the parchment sheets) to the baking sheet.
6. Bake for 12•15 minutes, or until the crackers are lightly golden and crisp.
7. Allow the crackers to cool completely before breaking them into pieces.

For the Salsa:
1. In a medium bowl, combine the diced tomatoes, chopped onion, jalapeño (if using), cilantro, lime juice, and salt. Stir to mix well.

Serve the whole grain crackers with the fresh salsa. Enjoy!

Tips:
• For a gluten•free version, use a gluten•free flour blend instead of whole wheat flour.
• Adjust the spiciness of the salsa by adding more or less jalapeño.
• Store any leftover crackers in an airtight container at room temperature for up to 1 week. Refrigerate the salsa in an airtight container for up to 3 days.

88. Energy Bites (made with dates and nuts)

Ingredient:

• 1 cup raw nuts (such as almonds, cashews, or walnuts)
• 1 cup pitted Medjool dates
• 2 tablespoons unsweetened shredded coconut (optional)
• 1 tablespoon chia seeds or ground flaxseed (optional)
• 1/4 teaspoon ground cinnamon (optional)
• Pinch of salt (optional)

Instructions:

1. In a food processor, pulse the raw nuts until they are finely chopped, but not turned into a butter.

2. Add the pitted Medjool dates to the food processor and pulse until the mixture starts to stick together.

3. If using, add the shredded coconut, chia seeds or flaxseed, cinnamon, and a pinch of salt. Pulse a few more times to incorporate.

4. Scoop the mixture by the tablespoonful and roll into bite•sized balls with your hands.

5. Place the energy bites on a parchment•lined baking sheet or plate.

6. Refrigerate the energy bites for at least 30 minutes to help them firm up.

7. Store the energy bites in an airtight container in the refrigerator for up to 1 week.

Tips:

• Use a variety of nuts to change up the flavor and texture.
• Dates provide natural sweetness, while the nuts offer healthy fats and protein.
• Avoid using any added sugars, oils, or other ingredients that may be difficult to digest for those without a gallbladder.
• Adjust the amount of coconut, seeds, or spices based on your personal preferences.
• These energy bites make a great portable snack or pre•workout fuel.

Enjoy these simple, gallbladder•friendly energy bites made with wholesome ingredients!

89. Dried Fruit

Ingredient:

• Assorted fresh fruit (such as apples, pears, bananas, mango, pineapple, etc.)

Equipment:
• Dehydrator or oven

Instructions:

Using a Dehydrator:
1. Wash and prepare the fruit:
  • Peel and slice the fruit into thin, even pieces, about 1/4•inch thick.
  • Remove any seeds, pits, or cores.

2. Arrange the fruit slices in a single layer on the dehydrator trays, making sure the slices are not overlapping.

3. Dehydrate the fruit at 135°F (57°C) for 8•12 hours, or until the fruit is dried and leathery in texture. The exact time may vary depending on the type of fruit and your dehydrator.

4. Once dried, allow the fruit to cool completely before storing.

Using an Oven:
1. Preheat your oven to the lowest temperature setting, usually around 135°F (57°C).

2. Prepare the fruit as described above for the dehydrator method.

3. Line baking sheets with parchment paper and arrange the fruit slices in a single layer.

4. Bake the fruit for 8•12 hours, flipping the slices occasionally, until they are dried and leathery.

5. Turn off the oven and leave the fruit inside to cool completely before removing.

Storage:
1. Once the dried fruit has cooled, store it in an airtight container at room temperature.

2. Properly dried fruit can be stored for up to 1 year, depending on the type of fruit.

90. Rice Paper Spring Rolls

Ingredient:

• 8•10 rice paper wrappers
• 1 cup shredded cabbage or lettuce
• 1 cup julienned carrots
• 1 cup julienned cucumber
• 1/2 cup cooked and chilled rice noodles
• 1/4 cup fresh mint leaves
• 1/4 cup fresh cilantro leaves
• Dipping sauce (such as peanut sauce, hoisin sauce, or soy sauce)

Instructions:

1. Fill a shallow dish or pie plate with warm water. Dip one rice paper wrapper into the water, turning it to fully submerge it. Allow the wrapper to soak for 10•20 seconds until it becomes pliable.

2. Carefully transfer the softened wrapper to a clean, damp work surface.

3. In the center of the wrapper, layer a small amount of the shredded cabbage/lettuce, julienned carrots and cucumber, cooked rice noodles, mint leaves, and cilantro leaves.

4. Fold the bottom of the wrapper up over the filling, then fold in the sides and continue rolling tightly to enclose the filling.

5. Repeat the process with the remaining wrappers and fillings. Serve the spring rolls immediately with your desired dipping sauce on the side.

Tips:
• Work with one wrapper at a time, keeping the remaining wrappers covered to prevent them from drying out.

• Adjust the fillings to your taste preferences or use other vegetables like bean sprouts, shredded chicken, or shrimp.

• For a heartier roll, add a small amount of cooked quinoa or brown rice to the filling.

• Store any leftover spring rolls in the refrigerator, wrapped in damp paper towels, for up to 2 days.

91. Vegan Sushi Rolls

Ingredient:

- 1 cup short•grain sushi rice
- 2 tablespoons rice vinegar
- 1 tablespoon sugar
- 1/2 teaspoon salt
- 4•6 sheets of nori (seaweed sheets)
- Fillings (choose 2•3):
  - Avocado, sliced
  - Cucumber, julienned
  - Carrots, julienned
  - Cooked and chilled sweet potato, sliced
  - Marinated tofu, sliced
  - Shredded cabbage or lettuce
  - Mango, sliced
  - Cream cheese alternative (such as cashew•based)

Equipment: Bamboo sushi mat

Instructions:

1. Cook the sushi rice according to package instructions. Transfer to a large bowl and let cool slightly.

2. In a small bowl, mix together the rice vinegar, sugar, and salt. Pour this mixture over the warm rice and gently fold to combine. Allow the rice to cool completely.

3. Place a nori sheet shiny•side down on the bamboo sushi mat. Spread about 3/4 cup of the prepared sushi rice evenly over the nori, leaving a 1•inch border at the top.

4. Arrange your desired fillings in a line across the center of the rice.

5. Using the sushi mat, tightly roll the nori around the fillings, starting from the bottom and rolling towards the top. Moisten the top edge with water to seal the roll.

6. Slice the sushi roll into 6•8 pieces using a sharp, wet knife.

7. Repeat the rolling process with the remaining nori sheets and fillings.

8. Serve the vegan sushi rolls with soy sauce, wasabi, and pickled ginger, if desired.

92. Tofu Lettuce Wraps

Ingredient:

• 1 block (14 oz) firm or extra•firm tofu, drained and pressed
• 2 tablespoons soy sauce or tamari
• 1 tablespoon rice vinegar
• 1 teaspoon sesame oil
• 1 teaspoon grated ginger
• 1 garlic clove, minced
• 1/4 teaspoon red pepper flakes (optional)
• 1 cup shredded carrots
• 1 cup thinly sliced cucumber
• 1/2 cup thinly sliced red bell pepper
• 1/4 cup chopped green onions
• 12•16 large lettuce leaves (such as romaine, bibb, or butter lettuce)

For the Sauce (optional):
• 2 tablespoons peanut butter (or tahini)
• 2 tablespoons soy sauce or tamari
• 1 tablespoon rice vinegar
• 1 teaspoon sesame oil
• 1 teaspoon honey or maple syrup
• 1 tablespoon water

Instructions:

1. In a medium bowl, crumble the pressed tofu into small pieces.

2. In a small bowl, whisk together the soy sauce, rice vinegar, sesame oil, ginger, garlic, and red pepper flakes (if using). Pour this mixture over the crumbled tofu and gently toss to coat.

3. In a separate bowl, combine the shredded carrots, sliced cucumber, bell pepper, and green onions.

4. If making the optional sauce, whisk together all the sauce ingredients in a small bowl.

5. To assemble the wraps, place a lettuce leaf on a plate and top with a portion of the seasoned tofu and the vegetable mixture.

6. Drizzle the optional peanut sauce over the top, if desired. Fold the sides of the lettuce leaf over the filling and enjoy.

93. Jackfruit Tacos

Ingredient:

• 2 (20 oz) cans young green jackfruit, drained and shredded
• 1 tablespoon olive oil
• 1 onion, diced
• 3 garlic cloves, minced
• 1 tablespoon chili powder
• 1 teaspoon cumin
• 1 teaspoon smoked paprika
• 1/2 teaspoon oregano
• 1/4 teaspoon cayenne pepper (optional)
• 1 cup vegetable broth
• 2 tablespoons tomato paste
• Salt and pepper to taste
• 12•16 small corn or flour tortillas
• Toppings (such as diced avocado, shredded cabbage, diced onion, cilantro, lime wedges)

Instructions:

1. Drain and rinse the jackfruit. Use your hands or a fork to shred the jackfruit into a pulled pork•like texture.

2. In a large skillet, heat the olive oil over medium heat. Add the diced onion and sauté for 5•7 minutes until translucent.

3. Add the minced garlic and sauté for an additional minute until fragrant.

4. Stir in the shredded jackfruit, chili powder, cumin, smoked paprika, oregano, and cayenne (if using). Mix well to coat the jackfruit.

5. Pour in the vegetable broth and tomato paste. Bring the mixture to a simmer and cook for 15•20 minutes, stirring occasionally, until the jackfruit is tender and the liquid has reduced.

6. Season the jackfruit filling with salt and pepper to taste. Warm the tortillas according to package instructions.

7. To assemble the tacos, place a portion of the jackfruit filling into each tortilla. Top with your desired toppings. Serve the jackfruit tacos immediately, with any extra toppings on the side.

94. Vegan Cheese Platter with Crackers

Ingredient:

• 2•3 varieties of vegan cheese (such as cashew•based, nut•based, or coconut•based)
• Dried fruit (e.g., apricots, figs, dates)
• Fresh fruit (e.g., grapes, apple slices, pear slices)
• Nuts and seeds (e.g., almonds, walnuts, pumpkin seeds)
• Olives (optional)
• Cornichons or pickled vegetables (optional)
• Crackers or bread (gluten•free or whole grain)
• Honey or jam (optional)

Assembly Instructions:

1. Arrange the vegan cheese wedges or slices on a large serving platter or board.

2. Scatter the dried fruit, fresh fruit, nuts, and seeds around the cheese.

3. Add any optional items like olives or pickled vegetables.

4. Place the crackers or bread around the edges of the platter.

5. If desired, drizzle a small amount of honey or place a small bowl of jam next to the platter.

6. Serve the vegan cheese platter at room temperature.

Tips:

• Choose a variety of vegan cheese flavors and textures for a more interesting platter (e.g., soft, hard, spreadable).

• Slice or cube the vegan cheese to make it easier for guests to serve themselves.

• Arrange the items in a visually appealing way, using different colors and shapes.

• Provide small plates, napkins, and toothpicks or cheese knives for easy serving.

• Adjust the quantities based on the number of guests you're serving.

• Store any leftover vegan cheese and accompaniments separately in the refrigerator.

95. Stuffed Bell Peppers with Quinoa

Ingredient:

• 4 large bell peppers
• 1 cup quinoa
• 2 cups vegetable broth (low•fat or fat•free)
• 1 can (15 oz) black beans, drained and rinsed
• 1 can (15 oz) diced tomatoes (low•fat or no added fat)
• 1 cup corn kernels
• 1 small onion, diced
• 2 cloves garlic, minced
• 1 teaspoon cumin
• 1 teaspoon chili powder
• Salt and pepper to taste
• Nutritional yeast (optional, for a cheesy flavor)
• Fresh cilantro for garnish

Instructions:
1. Preheat the oven to 375°F (190°C).

2. Cut the tops off the bell peppers and remove the seeds and membranes. Place the peppers in a baking dish.

3. In a medium saucepan, combine quinoa and vegetable broth. Bring to a boil, then reduce heat, cover, and simmer for about 15 minutes, or until the quinoa is cooked and the liquid is absorbed.

4. In a large skillet, sauté the onion and garlic until softened. Add the black beans, diced tomatoes, corn, cumin, chili powder, salt, and pepper. Cook for a few minutes until heated through.

5. Add the cooked quinoa to the skillet and mix everything together.

6. Stuff the bell peppers with the quinoa mixture.

7. Sprinkle some nutritional yeast on top of each stuffed pepper for a cheesy flavor.

8. Cover the baking dish with foil and bake for about 25•30 minutes, or until the peppers are tender.

9. Remove the foil and bake for an additional 5•10 minutes. Garnish with fresh cilantro before serving.

96. Artichoke and Spinach Dip (vegan)

Ingredient:

• 1 can (14 oz) artichoke hearts, drained and chopped
• 1 cup frozen chopped spinach, thawed and drained
• 1 cup raw cashews, soaked in water for at least 2 hours or overnight
• 1/2 cup unsweetened almond milk
• 2 cloves garlic, minced
• 1/4 cup nutritional yeast
• 1 tablespoon lemon juice
• 1 teaspoon onion powder
• 1/2 teaspoon salt
• 1/4 teaspoon black pepper
• Pinch of red pepper flakes (optional)
• Fresh parsley for garnish

Instructions:

1. Preheat the oven to 350°F (175°C).

2. In a food processor or blender, combine the soaked cashews, almond milk, garlic, nutritional yeast, lemon juice, onion powder, salt, pepper, and red pepper flakes. Blend until smooth and creamy.

3. In a mixing bowl, combine the chopped artichoke hearts, chopped spinach, and the cashew cream mixture. Mix well to combine.

4. Transfer the mixture to a baking dish and spread it out evenly.

5. Bake for about 20•25 minutes, or until the dip is heated through and bubbly.

6. Remove from the oven and garnish with fresh parsley.

7. Serve the Artichoke and Spinach Dip warm with your favorite dippers such as tortilla chips, crackers, or sliced vegetables.

Enjoy this creamy and flavorful vegan Artichoke and Spinach Dip at your next gathering or as a tasty snack!

97. Zucchini Fritters

Ingredient:

• 2 medium zucchini, grated (about 2 cups)
• 1/2 cup all•purpose flour (or gluten•free flour blend)
• 2 eggs, lightly beaten
• 1/4 cup grated Parmesan cheese (or vegan Parmesan alternative)
• 2 tablespoons chopped fresh parsley
• 1 garlic clove, minced
• 1/2 teaspoon baking powder
• 1/4 teaspoon salt
• 1/4 teaspoon black pepper
• 2 tablespoons olive oil or avocado oil for frying

Instructions:

1. Grate the zucchini using a box grater or food processor. Place the grated zucchini in a clean kitchen towel or cheesecloth and squeeze out as much moisture as possible.

2. In a medium bowl, combine the grated and drained zucchini, flour, eggs, Parmesan, parsley, garlic, baking powder, salt, and pepper. Mix until well incorporated.

3. Heat the olive oil in a large skillet over medium heat.

4. Scoop heaping tablespoons of the zucchini mixture and gently place them in the hot oil, flattening them slightly with a spatula to form fritters.

5. Fry the zucchini fritters for 2•3 minutes per side, or until golden brown.

6. Transfer the cooked fritters to a paper towel•lined plate to drain any excess oil.

7. Serve the zucchini fritters warm, with your desired toppings or dipping sauces, such as:
   • Tzatziki or vegan yogurt sauce
   • Marinara or tomato sauce
   • Pesto

98. Vegan Caesar Salad

Ingredient:

For the Caesar Dressing:
• 1/2 cup raw cashews, soaked in water for at least 2 hours or overnight
• 2 tablespoons lemon juice
• 2 tablespoons nutritional yeast
• 1 tablespoon Dijon mustard
• 1 clove garlic, minced
• 1/4 cup water
• Salt and pepper to taste

For the Salad:
• 1 large head of romaine lettuce, chopped
• 1 cup cherry tomatoes, halved
• 1/2 cup croutons (look for low•fat or no added fat options)
• 1/4 cup sliced black olives
• 2 tablespoons capers (optional)
• Vegan parmesan cheese (optional)

Instructions:

1. To make the Caesar dressing, drain and rinse the soaked cashews. In a blender, combine the cashews, lemon juice, nutritional yeast, Dijon mustard, garlic, water, salt, and pepper. Blend until smooth and creamy. Add more water if needed to reach your desired consistency. Set aside.

2. In a large salad bowl, combine the chopped romaine lettuce, cherry tomatoes, black olives, and capers.

3. Add the Caesar dressing to the salad and toss until well coated.

4. Top the salad with croutons and vegan parmesan cheese, if desired.

5. Serve the Vegan Caesar Salad immediately and enjoy!

This vegan Caesar Salad is light, flavorful, and gallbladder•friendly. It's a delicious and healthy option for a satisfying meal or side dish.

99. Portobello Mushroom Burger

Ingredient:

• 4 large bell peppers
• 1 cup quinoa
• 2 cups vegetable broth
• 1 can (15 oz) black beans, drained and rinsed
• 1 can (15 oz) diced tomatoes
• 1 cup corn kernels
• 1 small onion, diced
• 2 cloves garlic, minced
• 1 teaspoon cumin
• 1 teaspoon chili powder
• Salt and pepper to taste
• 1 cup shredded cheese (optional)
• Fresh cilantro for garnish

Instructions:
1. Preheat the oven to 375°F (190°C).

2. Cut the tops off the bell peppers and remove the seeds and membranes. Place the peppers in a baking dish.

3. In a medium saucepan, combine quinoa and vegetable broth. Bring to a boil, then reduce heat, cover, and simmer for about 15 minutes, or until the quinoa is cooked and the liquid is absorbed.

4. In a large skillet, sauté the onion and garlic until softened. Add the black beans, diced tomatoes, corn, cumin, chili powder, salt, and pepper. Cook for a few minutes until heated through.

5. Add the cooked quinoa to the skillet and mix everything together.

6. Stuff the bell peppers with the quinoa mixture. If desired, top each pepper with shredded cheese.

7. Cover the baking dish with foil and bake for about 25•30 minutes, or until the peppers are tender.

8. Remove the foil and bake for an additional 5•10 minutes to melt the cheese. Garnish with fresh cilantro before serving.

100. Ratatouille

Ingredient:

- 1 eggplant, diced
- 2 zucchinis, diced
- 1 yellow bell pepper, diced
- 1 red bell pepper, diced
- 1 onion, diced
- 3 cloves garlic, minced
- 1 can (15 oz) diced tomatoes
- 2 tablespoons tomato paste
- 1 teaspoon dried thyme
- 1 teaspoon dried oregano
- Salt and pepper to taste
- Fresh basil for garnish
- Olive oil for cooking

Instructions:

1. In a large skillet or pot, heat some olive oil over medium heat.

2. Add the diced onion and garlic, and sauté until softened.

3. Add the diced eggplant, zucchinis, and bell peppers to the skillet. Cook for about 5•7 minutes, or until the vegetables start to soften.

4. Stir in the diced tomatoes, tomato paste, dried thyme, dried oregano, salt, and pepper. Mix well to combine.

5. Cover the skillet and let the Ratatouille simmer over low heat for about 20•25 minutes, stirring occasionally, until the vegetables are tender.

6. Adjust the seasoning with more salt and pepper if needed.

7. Serve the Ratatouille hot, garnished with fresh basil.

This vegan Ratatouille is a flavorful and comforting dish that is gentle on the digestive system and suitable for those without a gallbladder. Enjoy it as a main dish or as a side with crusty bread or over cooked grains like quinoa or rice.

101. Fresh herbs/spices

Ingredient:

- 1 cup fresh parsley, finely chopped
- 1/4 cup fresh cilantro, finely chopped
- 3 cloves garlic, minced
- 1/4 cup red wine vinegar
- 1/2 cup olive oil
- 1 tablespoon fresh oregano, chopped (or 1 teaspoon dried oregano)
- 1/2 teaspoon red pepper flakes (adjust to taste)
- Salt and pepper to taste

Instructions:

1. In a bowl, combine the chopped parsley, cilantro, garlic, red wine vinegar, olive oil, oregano, and red pepper flakes.

2. Mix well to combine all the ingredients.

3. Season with salt and pepper to taste. Adjust the seasoning as needed.

4. Let the Chimichurri Sauce sit for at least 30 minutes to allow the flavors to meld together.

5. Serve the Chimichurri Sauce as a condiment for grilled meats, roasted vegetables, or as a dipping sauce for bread.

Chimichurri Sauce is a versatile and delicious addition to many dishes, adding a burst of fresh herb and tangy flavor. Enjoy this zesty sauce with your favorite meals!

102. Vegan mayonnaise

Ingredient:

• 1/2 cup unsweetened soy milk or almond milk
• 1 cup vegetable oil
• 1 tablespoon apple cider vinegar or lemon juice
• 1 teaspoon Dijon mustard
• 1/2 teaspoon salt
• 1/2 teaspoon sugar (optional)
• Pinch of ground turmeric (for color, optional)

Instructions:

1. In a blender or food processor, combine the soy milk, apple cider vinegar or lemon juice, Dijon mustard, salt, sugar, and turmeric.

2. Blend the ingredients on low speed until well combined.

3. While the blender is running, slowly drizzle in the vegetable oil in a thin stream. This will help emulsify the mixture and create a creamy consistency.

4. Continue blending until the mixture thickens and resembles the texture of mayonnaise.

5. Taste the vegan mayonnaise and adjust the seasoning if needed by adding more salt, sugar, or lemon juice.

6. Transfer the vegan mayonnaise to a jar or container and store it in the refrigerator. It will thicken further as it chills.

This homemade Vegan Mayonnaise is a great dairy•free alternative to traditional mayonnaise and can be used in sandwiches, salads, dressings, and dips. Enjoy the creamy texture and tangy flavor of this plant•based condiment!

103. Oatmeal raisin cookies

Ingredient:

- 1 cup all•purpose flour
- 1 teaspoon baking soda
- 1 teaspoon ground cinnamon
- 1/2 teaspoon salt
- 1/2 cup coconut oil, melted
- 1/2 cup brown sugar
- 1/4 cup granulated sugar
- 1 flax egg (1 tablespoon ground flaxseed + 3 tablespoons water)
- 1 teaspoon vanilla extract
- 1 1/2 cups old•fashioned oats
- 1/2 cup raisins

Instructions:

1. Preheat the oven to 350°F (175°C) and line a baking sheet with parchment paper.

2. In a small bowl, prepare the flax egg by mixing the ground flaxseed with water. Let it sit for a few minutes to thicken.

3. In a medium bowl, whisk together the flour, baking soda, cinnamon, and salt.

4. In a large bowl, mix the melted coconut oil, brown sugar, and granulated sugar until well combined.

5. Add the flax egg and vanilla extract to the wet ingredients and mix until smooth.

6. Gradually add the dry ingredients to the wet ingredients, stirring until just combined.

7. Fold in the oats and raisins until evenly distributed in the dough.

8. Using a cookie scoop or spoon, drop rounded tablespoons of dough onto the prepared baking sheet, spacing them a few inches apart.

9. Bake for 10•12 minutes, or until the edges are golden brown.

10. Allow the cookies to cool on the baking sheet for a few minutes before transferring them to a wire rack to cool completely.

104. Homemade granola bars

Ingredient:

• 2 cups rolled oats
• 1/2 cup almond butter (or any nut or seed butter of your choice)
• 1/3 cup maple syrup or agave nectar
• 1/4 cup chopped nuts (such as almonds, walnuts, or pecans)
• 1/4 cup dried fruit (such as raisins, cranberries, or chopped dates)
• 1/4 cup pumpkin seeds or sunflower seeds
• 1/4 cup shredded coconut
• 1 teaspoon vanilla extract
• 1/2 teaspoon cinnamon
• Pinch of salt

Instructions:

1. Preheat the oven to 350°F (175°C) and line a baking dish with parchment paper.

2. In a large bowl, combine the rolled oats, chopped nuts, dried fruit, pumpkin seeds, shredded coconut, cinnamon, and salt.

3. In a small saucepan, heat the almond butter and maple syrup over low heat, stirring until well combined.

4. Remove the almond butter mixture from heat and stir in the vanilla extract.

5. Pour the almond butter mixture over the dry ingredients and mix well to combine.

6. Press the mixture firmly into the prepared baking dish, ensuring it is evenly spread and compacted.

7. Bake for about 20•25 minutes, or until the edges are golden brown.

8. Allow the granola bars to cool completely in the pan before cutting into bars.

These Homemade Vegan Granola Bars are a nutritious and delicious snack option that is gentle on the digestive system and suitable for those without a gallbladder. Enjoy these homemade bars as a convenient and satisfying treat on the go!

105. Veggie spring rolls

Ingredient:

For the Spring Rolls:
• Rice paper wrappers
• 1 cup cooked rice noodles
• 1 cup shredded lettuce
• 1 cucumber, julienned
• 1 carrot, julienned
• 1 bell pepper, thinly sliced
• Fresh herbs (such as mint, cilantro, and basil)
• Optional add•ins: tofu, avocado, bean sprouts

For the Dipping Sauce:
• 1/4 cup soy sauce or tamari
• 2 tablespoons rice vinegar
• 1 tablespoon maple syrup or agave nectar
• 1 clove garlic, minced
• 1 teaspoon grated ginger
• Red pepper flakes (optional)

Instructions:

1. Prepare all the veggies and herbs by cutting them into thin strips or julienne.

2. Fill a shallow dish with warm water. Dip one rice paper wrapper into the water for a few seconds until it softens.

3. Place the softened rice paper wrapper on a clean surface.

4. Layer a small amount of cooked rice noodles, shredded lettuce, cucumber, carrot, bell pepper, fresh herbs, and any optional add•ins in the center of the rice paper wrapper.

5. Fold the sides of the wrapper over the filling, then roll it up tightly.

6. Repeat with the remaining ingredients to make more spring rolls.

7. In a small bowl, whisk together the ingredients for the dipping sauce until well combined. Serve the Veggie Spring Rolls with the dipping sauce on the side.

These Veggie Spring Rolls are light, refreshing, and packed with fresh vegetables, making them a healthy and gallbladder•friendly option for a light meal or snack. Enjoy the colorful and flavorful combination of veggies wrapped in rice paper!

106. Vegetable sushi

Ingredient:

• 2 cups sushi rice
• 2 1/2 cups water
• 1/3 cup rice vinegar
• 2 tablespoons sugar
• 1 teaspoon salt
• Nori seaweed sheets
• Assorted vegetables for filling (such as cucumber, avocado, carrot, bell pepper, and tofu)
• Soy sauce, pickled ginger, and wasabi for serving

Instructions:

1. Rinse the sushi rice under cold water until the water runs clear. Combine the rice and water in a rice cooker or pot and cook according to the package instructions.

2. In a small saucepan, combine the rice vinegar, sugar, and salt. Heat over low heat until the sugar and salt dissolve. Remove from heat and let it cool.

3. Once the rice is cooked, transfer it to a large bowl and gently fold in the vinegar mixture to season the rice. Let the rice cool to room temperature.

4. Prepare your vegetables by cutting them into thin strips or julienne.

5. Place a sheet of nori on a bamboo sushi mat. Wet your hands and spread a thin layer of sushi rice over the nori, leaving a small border at the top.

6. Arrange your vegetable fillings in a line across the center of the rice.

7. Roll the sushi tightly using the bamboo mat, applying gentle pressure as you roll.

8. Wet the border of the nori sheet with a little water to seal the roll.

9. Use a sharp knife to slice the sushi roll into individual pieces.

10. Serve the vegetable sushi with soy sauce, pickled ginger, and wasabi on the side.

Enjoy this delicious and healthy Vegan Vegetable Sushi that is gentle on the digestive system and suitable for those without a gallbladder.

107. Baked veggie chips

Ingredient:

- Assorted vegetables (such as sweet potatoes, beets, zucchini, carrots, or kale)
- Olive oil
- Salt and pepper
- Optional seasonings: garlic powder, paprika, cumin, or nutritional yeast

Instructions:

1. Preheat the oven to 375°F (190°C) and line a baking sheet with parchment paper.

2. Wash and peel the vegetables (if needed) and slice them thinly using a mandoline slicer or a sharp knife.

3. Place the sliced vegetables in a bowl and drizzle with olive oil. Toss to coat the vegetables evenly.

4. Season the vegetables with salt, pepper, and any optional seasonings of your choice. Mix well to ensure the seasonings are evenly distributed.

5. Arrange the seasoned vegetable slices in a single layer on the prepared baking sheet.

6. Bake in the preheated oven for about 15•20 minutes, or until the chips are crispy and lightly browned. Keep an eye on them to prevent burning.

7. Remove the baking sheet from the oven and let the veggie chips cool slightly before serving.

These Baked Veggie Chips are a healthy and flavorful snack alternative to store•bought chips. They are low in fat and can be customized with your favorite seasonings. Enjoy these crispy and nutritious chips as a guilt•free snack or side dish!

108. Roasted chickpeas

Ingredient:

• 1 can (15 oz) chickpeas (garbanzo beans), drained and rinsed
• 1•2 tablespoons olive oil
• 1 teaspoon ground cumin
• 1 teaspoon paprika
• 1/2 teaspoon garlic powder
• 1/2 teaspoon onion powder
• Salt and pepper to taste

Instructions:

1. Preheat the oven to 400°F (200°C) and line a baking sheet with parchment paper.

2. Pat the chickpeas dry with a paper towel to remove excess moisture.

3. In a bowl, toss the chickpeas with olive oil, cumin, paprika, garlic powder, onion powder, salt, and pepper until evenly coated.

4. Spread the seasoned chickpeas in a single layer on the prepared baking sheet.

5. Roast in the preheated oven for about 25•30 minutes, shaking the pan halfway through, until the chickpeas are crispy and golden brown.

6. Remove from the oven and let the roasted chickpeas cool slightly before serving.

These Roasted Chickpeas are a crunchy and protein•packed snack that can be enjoyed on their own, added to salads for extra texture, or used as a topping for soups and bowls. Experiment with different seasonings to customize the flavor to your liking. Enjoy these tasty and nutritious roasted chickpeas!

109. Edamame salad

Ingredient:

- 2 cups shelled edamame (fresh or frozen, thawed)
- 1 red bell pepper, diced
- 1/2 cucumber, diced
- 1/4 cup red onion, finely chopped
- 1/4 cup fresh cilantro, chopped
- 2 tablespoons sesame seeds
- 2 tablespoons rice vinegar
- 1 tablespoon soy sauce or tamari
- 1 tablespoon sesame oil
- 1 tablespoon maple syrup or agave nectar
- 1 clove garlic, minced
- Salt and pepper to taste

Instructions:

1. In a large bowl, combine the shelled edamame, diced red bell pepper, diced cucumber, chopped red onion, and chopped cilantro.

2. In a small bowl, whisk together the rice vinegar, soy sauce, sesame oil, maple syrup, minced garlic, salt, and pepper to make the dressing.

3. Pour the dressing over the edamame salad and toss to coat the ingredients evenly.

4. Sprinkle sesame seeds over the salad and gently mix them in.

5. Chill the Edamame Salad in the refrigerator for at least 30 minutes to allow the flavors to meld together.

6. Serve the salad chilled as a refreshing and nutritious side dish or light meal.

This Edamame Salad is a flavorful and protein•packed dish that is perfect for a quick and healthy meal. Enjoy the combination of crunchy vegetables, nutty edamame, and savory dressing in this delicious salad!

110. Black bean brownies

Ingredient:

• 1 can (15 oz) black beans, drained and rinsed
• 3 tablespoons coconut oil, melted
• 1/2 cup cocoa powder
• 1/4 teaspoon salt
• 1 teaspoon vanilla extract
• 1/2 cup sugar (you can adjust the amount to your preference)
• 2 flax eggs (2 tablespoons ground flaxseed + 6 tablespoons water)
• 1/2 teaspoon baking powder
• 1/2 cup chocolate chips (optional)

Instructions:

1. Preheat the oven to 350°F (175°C) and grease a baking pan.

2. Prepare the flax eggs by mixing the ground flaxseed with water in a small bowl. Let it sit for a few minutes to thicken.

3. In a food processor, combine the black beans, melted coconut oil, cocoa powder, salt, vanilla extract, sugar, flax eggs, and baking powder. Blend until smooth and well combined.

4. Fold in the chocolate chips, if using.

5. Pour the batter into the prepared baking pan and spread it out evenly.

6. Bake for about 20•25 minutes, or until a toothpick inserted into the center comes out clean.

7. Allow the brownies to cool before slicing and serving.

These Black Bean Brownies are a healthier alternative to traditional brownies, as they are packed with fiber and protein from the black beans. Enjoy this delicious and nutritious treat!

III. Vegan energy bites

Ingredient:

- 1 cup rolled oats
- 1/2 cup almond butter (or any nut or seed butter of your choice)
- 1/3 cup maple syrup or agave nectar
- 1/4 cup ground flaxseed
- 1/4 cup shredded coconut
- 1 teaspoon vanilla extract
- 1/2 cup chopped nuts (such as almonds, walnuts, or pecans)
- 1/4 cup dried fruit (such as raisins, cranberries, or chopped dates)
- Pinch of salt

Instructions:

1. In a large mixing bowl, combine the rolled oats, almond butter, maple syrup, ground flaxseed, shredded coconut, vanilla extract, chopped nuts, dried fruit, and a pinch of salt.

2. Mix all the ingredients together until well combined. If the mixture is too dry, you can add a little more almond butter or maple syrup to help bind everything together.

3. Once the mixture is well combined, use your hands to roll the mixture into small bite•sized balls.

4. Place the energy bites on a baking sheet lined with parchment paper and refrigerate for at least 30 minutes to set.

5. Store the Vegan Energy Bites in an airtight container in the refrigerator for up to a week.

These Vegan Energy Bites are a great snack option for those without a gallbladder, as they are easy to digest and provide a quick boost of energy. Enjoy these tasty and nutritious bites throughout the day!

Navigating life without a gallbladder while adhering to a vegan diet may have seemed daunting at first, but by embracing the guidance and recipes in the ***"No Gallbladder Diet Cookbook for Vegans: Rebalance and Revitalize for Sensitive Digestion After Gallbladder Removal with 110+ Recipes Over 90 Days,"*** you have made significant strides towards improving your digestive health and overall well-being.

Celebrating Your Progress

Over the past 90 days, you have embarked on a journey to rebalance and revitalize your digestive system. By choosing plant-based, easy-to-digest foods, you have provided your body with the nutrients it needs to adapt to its new normal. This commitment to your health is commendable and has likely resulted in noticeable improvements in your digestion, energy levels, and overall vitality.

Continuing Your Healthy Lifestyle

While the 90-day plan has laid a solid foundation, maintaining these healthy habits is essential for long-term well-being. Here are some key points to keep in mind as you move forward:

- ***Stay Versatile:*** Continue to explore new recipes and ingredients that align with your dietary needs. Variety will keep your meals exciting and nutritionally balanced.

- ***Listen to Your Body:*** Pay close attention to how your body responds to different foods. This mindfulness will help you make adjustments as needed to maintain digestive comfort.

- ***Stay Educated:*** Keep learning about nutrition and digestive health. Staying informed will empower you to make the best choices for your body.

- ***Incorporate Other Healthy Habits:*** Combine your diet with regular physical activity, adequate hydration, and stress management techniques to further enhance your overall health.

Thank you for entrusting us with your health journey. Here's to a future filled with delicious vegan meals, improved digestion, and renewed vitality!